SET IT
FORGET IT

SET IT
FORGET IT

DANIEL ERICHSEN

ACKNOWLEDGEMENTS

There's nobody on the planet that has helped me more in making this book happen than my wife Jamie Rabot. Not only by being her kind and supportive self but also by teaching me how the mind works and by designing all the illustrations. Thank you for everything.

LA, who drew all the illustrations, I'm so happy having your work here. I believe it will truly change the experience of reading this book for which I'm ever grateful.

Nick Wignall, thank you for teaching me how perfectly the expression set it and forget it applies to sleep and giving me a name for this book. I hope it will not dissuade you from writing another one with me one day.

Michael Schwartz and Martin Reed, thank you for all your insights and support. Every path is easier when you know you're not alone.

Last but certainly not least, a huge thank you to anyone from the YouTube community that has ever left a comment or sent me an email. I have learned more from you than from any other source and I know you have so much more to teach me.

INSTRUCTIONS

Hi there!

I'm super excited that you've decided to use Set it & Forget it to get past your insomnia and to a place of amazing sleep!

Speaking of your destination, here's something that will help you get there.

Remember it's not a race. Getting to the last page in 6 hours does not mean you'll start sleeping fantastic. Understanding every chapter on the other hand will! And that may take some time.

Set away a minute after each chapter to think about what you just read. Does it make sense? Do you have any reservations? Are you ready to move forward?

Your goal after completing part one, Set it, is to understand what insomnia is and why you've had trouble sleeping.

When you reach part two, Forget it, your goal becomes to start shifting attention away from sleep. Slow down on the reading. Do more of things you enjoy and perhaps have postponed until you're sleeping better.

If you come across anything you're not sure makes sense, read the chapter one more time. Use my YouTube channel/Podcast The Sleep Coach School to your advantage. All the material in this book is explained and contextualized in hundreds of hours of free content. This includes me using Set it & Forget it when answering questions or talking with people who've had trouble sleeping just like you.

If you're still not sure, please leave a comment on the YouTube channel or head to www.thesleepcoachschool.com and use the form for questions to be answered in Open class. These are videos where myself or other coaches answer questions in live episodes.

With that said, we are ready to move ahead and start learning. Before we do, I want to thank you for giving me this chance to help you sleep better.

Sincerely,
Daniel

SET iT

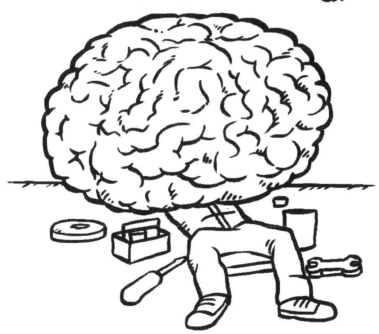

If you've had trouble sleeping for a few weeks or months, you may feel that this chapter doesn't apply to you. And that's right. It was indeed written to make sure someone with long time sleep issues is ready for change. This said, you can still learn something very important so do stick around!

If you on the other hand have struggled for years or even decades, then it is very important that you ask yourself how you feel about getting better.

Yes that's right. It is important that you ask yourself how you feel about getting better.

The obvious reason you may be surprised to read these lines is - who wouldn't want to sleep better?

Here's the thing - having insomnia for years does things to you that you may not be consciously aware of.

Firstly, the process of trying to figure out why you're not sleeping and trying to find things that could make you sleep year after year can affect your identity. You may start thinking of yourself as an insomniac.

You may feel that having trouble sleeping is part of who you are. This can lead to a place where thinking of yourself as someone who sleeps well seems foreign. It's hard to change your identity.

Secondly, all the time and effort spent on sleep can feel like an investment. Was all the pondering, all the experimenting and all the preoccupation really for nothing?

It can be difficult to accept that all the things you did to sleep better was no investment, but actually a big part of the problem.

Thirdly, having insomnia can let you off the hook. It is something to point to as the reason for why you are not doing things you've meant or wanted to do. It can be comforting to have something to blame for your shortcomings.

Finally, being the person that sleeps very little may give you attention as well as empathy which are both nice to get from friends and family.

Now take a look within. Ask yourself if you're holding on to insomnia for any reason. When you do, one of two things happen:

Either you find that the answer is no. And that's great! Nothing is standing in the way of you getting better sleep.

Or you find that you do take comfort in having insomnia at some level. It has served a purpose for you. And that's good too.

Because if you've identified a holdout, a recess in the brain that in fact is not ready to leave insomnia behind, well then you have something to work on.

It may not seem like much, but understanding that you may not have been ready in the past is the key to becoming fully committed to sleeping well now.

And when you are fully committed to a method that combines education and habit change - you will leave insomnia behind forever!

WHAT IS NORMAL SLEEP?

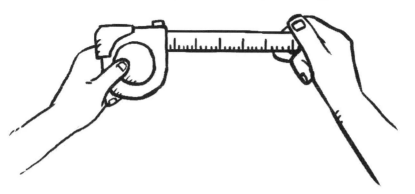

Do you remember a time when sleep was not a struggle? If you do then let that work in your favor. However you slept and felt back then is your reference point. That's the place you will get back to when you no longer worry about sleep.

If you can't remember a time when you didn't struggle to sleep, well then you don't have a reference point. Rather, you will learn as you move forward what sleeping well means to you.

Whether you have a reference point or not, knowing how most people sleep is important. Because from what you hear, you may think everyone but yourself is getting 8 hours of solid sleep every night. And feeling that you're way off an unattainable mark will not help you sleep any better. Well guess what, people sleep very differently from what we are told is ideal.

If you were to ask a bunch of people how much they sleep, they would say about 7 hours. Studies show that when healthy adults with no sleep problems are asked, their belief is that they get 7 hours of sleep.

In reality, most people don't have a clue.

Either they simply guess that they sleep about 7 hours because it sounds about right or they'll assume that they sleep 7 hours because they go to bed at 11 pm and get up at 6 am. When you objectively examine these same people, a different story emerges. Using electroencephalography (EEG) or actigraphy (think Fitbit) you find that their average sleep is actually a bit above 6 hours. Objectively measured, most adults sleep between 5.5 and 7 hours.

In other words, people with no trouble sleeping overestimate how much they sleep by about 1 hour. When we look at quality instead of quantity, things are very similar. Those without sleep problems believe they don't wake up during the night or only wake up a few times. In fact, when you study someone in the sleep lab, seeing a couple of awakenings every hour is the norm.

Again, most don't have a clue this is going on. They wake up multiple times but fall back asleep quickly and don't remember all the times they were awake during the night.

The problem here becomes that people paint a picture of how they sleep that isn't real. And this picture can make you feel as if you're just hopelessly displaced from "normal". You're not.

In this problem however, you can already start seeing the solution. Those people who sleep so great don't actually sleep so great. They paint a picture that isn't true, but they have no clue about that. Because they aren't paying any attention. And that's where you're heading as well.

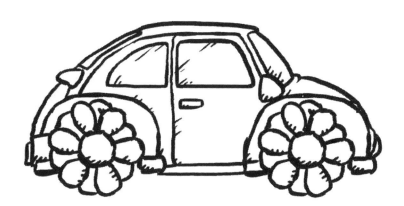

THE GAS AND THE BRAKE

Few things have been so mystified as sleep and insomnia. It is easy to get the impression that thousands of factors, many of which you can modify, control how well you sleep. The noise level, exposure to light, how much you ate, what time you ate, how much protein there was, what you did the hour before bedtime etc etc.

And this - the belief that multiple factors play an important role when it comes to your sleep, creates a ton of anxiety for no good reason.

If you're not sleeping well, then there must be one of a myriad of things that you're not getting right. You just have to figure out which one it is and tweak it. Alas, you tweaked the wrong thing and slept no better. Or you think you did but you aren't really sure. And now not knowing what you did to sleep better is making you more anxious. And lose more sleep. Here's the thing - sleep is not complicated.

In fact sleep is super simple. There are only two factors that determine how well you sleep, the gas and the brake. Let's start exploring this model by talking about appetite which just like sleep is a very simple system.

Ask yourself what you need to do to become hungry. Think about it for a second. What potion or ritual do you use to make yourself eat?

That's right. You become hungry even if you don't do anything in particular.

Now even though you don't have to do anything to become hungry, that doesn't mean there is no underlying biological process that is making you want to eat. In fact one thing and one thing only can produce hunger - and that's fasting.

Not eating is the only thing that makes you want to eat. And the longer you go without food, the stronger that urge becomes and the more you'll eventually end up eating.This said, hunger is not the only thing that determines how much you eat.

Imagine that you're really hungry, you feel you could eat anything put in front of you. But guess what, the only thing available is aged blue cheese which you can't stand. One whiff and just like that your appetite has evaporated.

And here you have it, the gas and brake model applied to eating. Your gas pedal is hunger and your brake pedal is negative emotion. The longer you go without eating the more gas you have in the system. The more negative emotion you have, related or unrelated to any particular food item, the more that brake pedal is pushed down.

This is exactly how sleep works as well. The one thing that can produce sleepiness, and sleep, is staying awake. However, even if you have a solid sleep drive, if you've been awake for a long period of time and feel sleepy, that sleepiness can disappear if you're anxious, worried or preoccupied.

Sleepiness, or sleep drive, is the gas in the sleep system. The longer you've been awake the stronger your sleep drive is and the more your body wants to sleep.

Hyperarousal (any type of heightened alertness such as stress, anxiety or excitement) is the brake in the sleep system.

That's it. This is how simple sleep is. Gas and Brake.

Take a minute to digest this and think about how all the things you've done to produce sleep has affected your sleep system. Have they increased your sleep drive, or have they increased your hyperarousal. Have you been hitting the gas pedal, brake pedal or both?

Once you're done reflecting, take a look at these four scenarios. Knowing that we have a gas pedal and brake pedal there are four combinations of gas and brake that will play out as follows when you go to bed:

> » No gas (not sleepy) and No brake (feeling relaxed) - In this scenario you will not sleep because your

sleep drive is not strong enough. However, this will not be a problem as you're relaxed. Think of this as resting peacefully.

- » No gas and Brake - In this scenario you definitely won't sleep at all. You don't have a sleep drive and you're hyperaroused. This is going to bed when you're wide awake and anxious.

- » Gas and Brake - This is a very common scenario. You are sleepy, but you are also hyperaroused. The hyperarousal is blocking you from sleeping.

- » Gas and No brake - This is where you want to be. You have a strong sleep drive and nothing that keeps it from sending you off to dreamland!

Having understood the above, knowing that there is no mystery and that in fact only two things determine how well you sleep, you have a great starting point to begin the work of setting it!

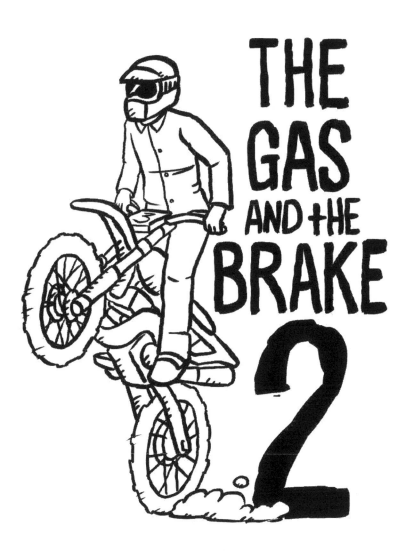

In the previous chapter we saw how the two things that determine how well we sleep are sleep drive (the gas) and hyperarousal (the brake). In this chapter, we will look at how to exploit this insight to sleep better. If you're not following, go back to the previous chapter and review. If something is still not clear, please send me a text or email!

A real practical way of using the gas and brake model is to explain what drives your insomnia. Because if you have trouble sleeping you either have a gas problem, a brake problem, or a combination of both. Let's take a look at which you have and what to do.

If you are not worried or preoccupied at all but find yourself spending a lot of time in bed not sleeping, you have a gas problem. You're in luck because it is pretty easy to get past!

Having a gas problem means that you're simply not sleepy enough when you go to bed or wake up from sleep. A common reason this happens is when someone decides to go to bed earlier to get more sleep. Your bedtime may have been 11 pm but you hear that you should get 8 hours of sleep and now go to bed 9 pm instead. You still end up falling asleep at around 11 pm but you're now spending 2 hours in bed without sleeping.

The solution to a gas problem is either to go to bed later or rise earlier. And just like that, a gas problem is fixed.

If you're not spending too much time in bed or sleeping during the day but rather, you are worried about your sleep, then you have a brake problem.

Brake problems require more work to get around but this is very doable. In fact pretty much everything you learn in this book will help with brake problems, the key being to shifting attention.

Here's the tricky part, deciding to take your foot off the brake pushes it down. Because anything you do with the intent of becoming less hyperaroused makes you more hyperaroused. In other words, anything you do to make yourself more calm makes you less calm.

Imagine that you've been anxious and decide to meditate to feel less anxious. Your intent is to become more calm. To see how well this is working your brain will monitor your anxiety levels closely. If you're not feeling more calm after 30 minutes, you'll continue for another 30. As you're meditating you'll wonder how much more meditation you'll have to do for it to start working. Your unwillingness to be anxious and the actions you take to become less anxious makes you more anxious.

The trick is to do something that channels your attention in a different direction. This could be anything that you do for fun and enjoyment.

If you like reading, that's great. If you prefer a Netflix show, perfect. Anything that you can do for pure pleasure is going to get the brake issue out of the way. This said, it will take time and you will learn much more as you keep reading this book that will get your foot away from the brake pedal.

Finally, if you are worried about sleep, if you catch sleep when you can, if you spend more than 6-7 hours in bed, you have both gas and brake problems. You're not sleepy enough when you go to bed and you're also hyperaroused. This is by far the most common. Almost everyone with trouble sleeping have a combination of gas and brake issues. And as you may guess from this, the solution lies in addressing both.

You need to both spend less time in bed AND shift attention away from sleep. You need to Set it & Forget it. And a great part to continue setting it is understanding why you have insomnia.

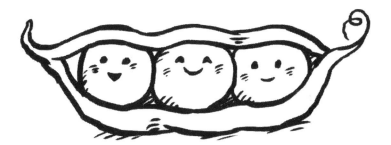

THIS IS WHY YOU HAVE INSOMNIA

One of the most important steps towards sleeping well is understanding how you ended up in a place of little sleep and lots of worries. Nothing explains this better than the 3 P model. Although the name may not spark a ton of curiosity, there is reason to be excited. Because once you understand how you got to where you are today, getting back to sleeping well is so much easier.

A quick note before we start - the more you can find things in this model that fit you the better. The belief that one's insomnia is unique and special is very common but not helpful. It leads to searching for a unique and special cure that doesn't exist. Finding things that fit on the other hand, starting to think of your insomnia as ordinary and typical, will lead you to a place of believing that you like countless others will sleep better when you Set it & Forget it. This said, let's start working!

1- Predisposition

Our first P is predisposing traits. Some of us are at baseline more likely to have trouble sleeping at some point in our lives. As we go through the four most common predisposing traits, ask yourself how these fit you.

» Having a type A personality, being a high achiever or perfectionist

» Having a tendency to worry

» Being an overthinker

» Being health conscious

If you have one or several of these traits, that's good! This means there's no mystery in terms of where your insomnia comes from. Also, you're the type of person who will do very well with the Set it & Forget it approach. Something else that is important to know is that there are millions of people who have all or many of these traits and sleep fantastic. It's helpful to know why you have trouble sleeping, and just as helpful to know that nothing is standing in your way of sleeping well.

So what do these traits have in common and why do they predispose you to having trouble sleeping?

The answer is attention.

You have the ability to focus your attention on a task, a thought or a concern and keep it there. Remember, that's an important ability! If you've done well in school and at work, you have your ability to focus to thank for your achievements. When it comes to sleep however, this otherwise amazing ability can work against you. Because attention is oxygen to insomnia, something it cannot survive without.

Here's the thing though, you can use your traits to work in your favor. If you're a high achiever, trying to achieve anything that is unrelated to sleep will help you tremendously. If you tend to obsess, obsess over anything but sleep and you'll sleep better.

If you don't have any of these four traits, then you're also in a great spot! You're not as predisposed to giving something sustained attention and that will serve you well.

2- Precipitating

Our second P is a precipitating event. It is a trigger that caused that initial bout of sleeplessness. You may immediately identify your precipitating event whether it was having a child, moving, going into menopause, a health scare or anything else. This trigger can be any event of increased stress or excitement that throws off your sleep.

It could also be that you don't find a specific precipitating event. Your trouble sleeping may have started more gradually over time.

Both having a clear precipitating event and not are common.

The thing that is most important to know is - not sleeping well after a stressful event is completely normal.

Imagine our ancestors living in bands of hunter-gatherers. If wolves were heard nearby, well then it would be very helpful to have less and more superficial sleep. When the wolves turned out to be a friendly tribe, then a return to good sleep would follow.

Or, to use another example, imagine that your friend just lost her job and went on to sleep great. That just doesn't sound right. We are supposed to sleep less in times of stress. Disrupted sleep is a completely normal and expected reaction.

It is the third P that is the problem, and the solution.

3- Perpetuating

So far, we have seen that being predisposed towards insomnia in itself is not a problem and that having disrupted sleep because of stress is expected. So far, everything is "normal". What happens next is what starts the process of developing ongoing insomnia from an episode of disturbed sleep - it is all about the reaction.

When you go through a stretch of nights with little sleep and start thinking of this as a problem, a spark is ignited.

The amygdala, the part of your brain that is to keep you out of harm's way, is now identifying lack of sleep as a threat, and starts treating sleeplessness the same way it does a charging bear. It tries to figure out what the threat is all about, it finds ways to try to fight it or escape it.

You may start by going to bed at the same time every night. Nope nothing changed. You then start keeping the bedroom dark. You're still not sleeping well. Something must be really wrong! You start wearing a sleep mask and playing soothing sounds at night, but nothing works.

As more and more things fail to make you sleep more, you feel that you must have a particularly severe case of insomnia which doesn't help you sleep any better. But what really is happening is the following:

Your amygdala is making you do things to eliminate the threat of sleeplessness. What it doesn't understand is that loss of sleep is not a bear, it's a perceived threat, none of all the things you're doing can produce sleep and it will appear as if nothing can fend off the threat. This kicks your amygdala into higher and higher gear. The higher the gear the more worried you become. The more worried the more things you try. The more you try the less you sleep. You get the point.

The process of trying to escape a perceived threat is what produces the illusion of a threat.

The behavior of problem solving is the problem.

Here's the good news - the insomnia cycle is completely reversible. The entire process can be put in rewind and you can get back to a place of good sleep. It may not be easy, but it is very doable. As you can tell from the 3 P model, the key to sleeping well is to give insomnia less attention and do less to produce sleep.

Understanding sleep efforts will take you a big step in that direction.

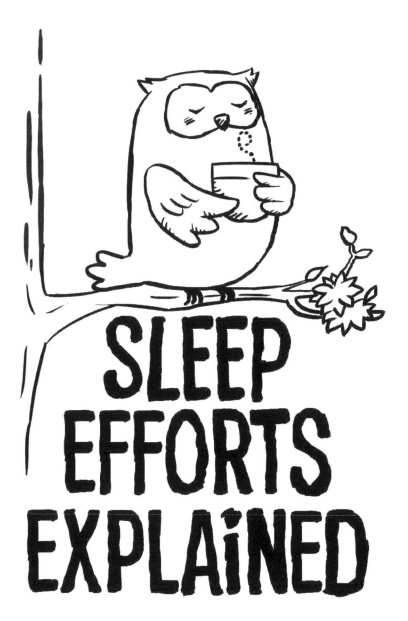

Here's something you're probably very familiar with that you didn't know had a name, a sleep effort. This is anything you do with the intent of producing more sleep. It's a very important concept to understand if you have trouble sleeping and look to change that.

Firstly, a bit of sleep physiology review. The only thing that can produce sleep is our sleep drive. Our bodies need for sleep. Our gas pedal. And the only thing that can create sleep drive is wakefulness. In a yin-yang type of way, the one thing that can produce sleep is wakefulness and the one thing that can produce wakefulness is sleep.

Here's the reason we are reviewing this again - knowing that only the act of staying awake can make you sleep, it's not hard to see that trying anything else is a recipe for trouble.

As a matter of fact, trying to change anything that is impossible to change is guaranteed to lead down a path of confusion and frustration. Try changing the weather or someone's opinion and you'll see.

The problem is, you didn't know until now that nothing but wakefulness can produce sleep, so you've tried a bunch of things.

Chances are that you've tried to produce sleep more than once and using more than one approach. You may have tried to use a supplement like melatonin or valerian root. You may have tried to keep the room dark and cool. You may have tried to read a boring book. These are all examples of sleep efforts.

Here's the thing, not only do sleep efforts not produce sleep, they produce insomnia. Either by taking you down the path of confusion, the path of frustration or both.

Let's say you tried valerian root and it "didn't work". Well then you feel worse, you probably have a severe case of insomnia. You're more worried and preoccupied, and you sleep less.

Let's say you tried valerian root and you slept better. It seems like it "worked" and you believe it produced sleep. Well now you're even worse off because your sleep confidence has started eroding. You have started believing that there is something inherently wrong with you and you need an outside source for sleep production. Your sleep has become vulnerable. Because when valerian root "stops working", you look for another outside sleep source in a never ending cycle of sleep efforts and eroding sleep confidence.

So what should you be doing?
If you aren't doing anything to produce sleep - well then that's fantastic and highly unusual, kudos to you! And just like the best way to stop smoking is to never start, you can simply avoid trying to produce sleep by external means.

If you after reading this realize that you have a lot of sleep efforts going on, the best thing to do is not necessarily stop them immediately, but start the process of questioning if they've helped you or not. Have they led you to build strong sleep confidence and consistently have good sleep or have they made you doubt your own ability to sleep? Was there a time when you took valerian root extract and you didn't sleep? Was there a time when you had a late coffee and slept well?

Have your sleep efforts helped you or hurt you?

HAVE THE RIGHT GOAL

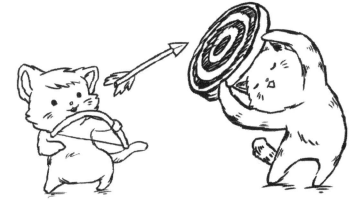

As opposed to many other journeys in life, when it comes to sleeping well, the destination is very important. You want to reach a place of peaceful sleep and leave the path to that place in the past. To do that, you have to have a goal that gives you direction rather than one that confuses your compass.

When you have trouble sleeping, one thing that appears very clear is that you're not getting enough sleep. Consequently, getting a certain amount of sleep can seem like a reasonable target. This could be 7 hours or 8 hours. Or it could be "the more the better".

In reality, this is the type of goal that leads you down a rabbit goal. And this is why:

An objective and measurable goal makes you become objective and measure your progress. To see how close you are to your goal of 7 hours you will check what time you went to bed and what time you got up. You will ask yourself how much you've slept or use a tracker to find this necessary information.

Here's the thing - starting to pay a lot of attention to your sleep is why you have insomnia, and now your goal is making you pay even more attention to your sleep.

And there's more.

As sleep can only be produced with wakefulness, all the things you do to get closer to your goal makes no difference. The amount you sleep doesn't budge no matter what you do. As your goal was to change your amount of sleep, you feel things are hopeless and frustrating. Feelings that don't help you at all.

You want to go in the complete opposite direction, you want a goal that is subjective and unmeasurable. Like feeling amazing. Or not worrying about sleep.

With a subjective and unmeasurable goal, you peel away attention from sleep. You start taking focus from the night to the day. You stop worrying about how many minutes it took you to fall asleep or what exact time you were up at night. On the contrary you note that you're feeling pretty good during the day and that you're stressing less about sleep.

You have a goal that serves you well.

THE SLEEP WINDOW

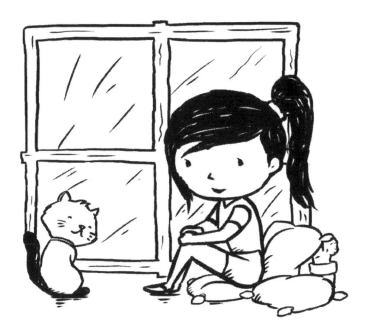

If you ask a bunch of insomnia therapists or coaches what the single most important thing to do is when having trouble sleeping, you're likely to get the same answer from most - spend less time in bed.

This may seem counter intuitive, you need more sleep, not less. And most people with insomnia try to compensate for little sleep over night by going to bed earlier and/or catching sleep when they can. As you may have experienced however, this doesn't get you to a place of great sleep. Even if you do sleep an extra hour in the morning or in the afternoon, you haven't taken a step towards sleeping well forever.

The opposite strategy on the other hand, spending less time in bed, will take you a big step towards fantastic sleep. And here's why:

1- Build a strong sleep drive

Remember the gas pedal? Remember how wakefulness is the only thing that can produce sleep? Well then you know that a strong sleep drive is important. By spending less time in bed, and more time in active wakefulness, that sleep drive grows stronger and helps you fall asleep, stay asleep and get better quality sleep.

2- Use reverse psychology

Insomnia comes from fear of losing sleep. The more you try to avoid sleeplessness, the more you train your brain that not sleeping is harmful and the stronger your fear of losing sleep becomes. In other words, wanting to sleep, pleading for sleep and trying to sleep are the reasons you're not sleeping.

Spending less time in bed is a super important psychological step away from trying to sleep.

When you spend less time in bed, you educate your brain that losing sleep is not a real threat. You teach it that it doesn't have to be afraid. You show it that it doesn't have to try so hard to make you sleep. And the less you try, the more you get.

3- Start believing

Typically, in the first 1-2 weeks of using a sleep window (if it takes longer for you, please know that's not unusual, you'll get there!) there is a moment when something unexpected happens. A positive surprise. You fell asleep easier than you thought you would. You fell back asleep pretty fast that time.

You didn't wake up at 3 am like you always do.

This may not initially seem like a big deal. But when it happens again, you realize that the strategy is working. This is the magical moment when you start believing that you CAN sleep, that there's nothing wrong with you and that you're on the right track.

Now that you know why you should spend less time in bed, the question becomes, how do you set a good sleep window?

Here's the thing, how much time you decide to spend in bed is much less important than that you don't question your decision and keep moving forward. For most people, spending about 7 hours in bed works great.

Also super important is that you have a consistent rise time.

More on why later.

For now, do this - ask yourself when a convenient time to get out of bed that you could stick to would be. Let's say that it's 6 am and that you've decided to spend 6.5 hours in bed. Well then you go 6.5 hours backwards from 6 am and you have your sleep window: 11:30 pm to 6 am. And here are your three goals:

Stay up until about 11:30 pm or later, even if you feel sleepy.

Get up around 6 am.

Don't sleep during the day.

Let's add a fourth one for good measure, if you're not sleepy at 11:30 pm, then it's not time to go to bed. Which begs the question, what should you do if you're not sleepy when your sleep window begins? Or in general for that matter, what type of bedtime routine should you have?

Well look at that, that happens to be exactly what we will talk about in our next chapter. Prepare for a surprise!

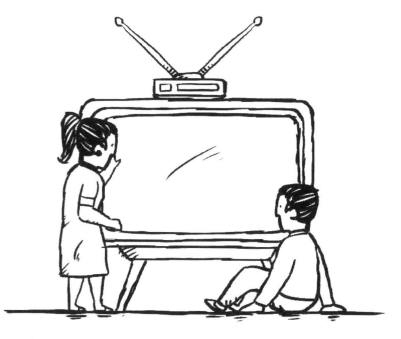

WHAT'S GOOD ON HULU?

You've probably heard that if you have trouble sleeping, it's important to create a good bedtime routine. You've been told to come up with a sequence of things to do before you go to bed that will maximize your chances of sleep. The problem here is that whomever came up with this idea put the cart before the horse. A relaxing bedtime routine is a consequence of sleeping well and not the other way around!

If you sleep well, then whatever you do before going to bed becomes a cue for sleep. If you're not sleeping well then whatever you do before going to bed becomes a cue for sleeplessness.

If you're excited about visiting your in law's then packing for that trip makes you feel happy. If you're dreading it, then the very same action of putting clothes in a bag makes you feel anxious. Your problem has nothing to do with how or what you're packing. If you know that, you can work on what really matters - your thoughts around the visit. When you've changed those and feel neutral or even positive about the trip, whatever you do in preparation will become a neutral or positive cue.

So doesn't it matter at all what you do before going to bed?

But yes it does matter! Because you can do a whole bunch of things that will make you sleep little. In fact you even know what these things are called...

...yes that's right. Sleep efforts!

Anything you do before going to bed with the intent of making yourself sleep more, whether it is meditating, taking a hot bath or avoiding screens will produce trouble sleeping.

So what should you do?

The answer is simple - it is of extreme importance that you do something you enjoy!

Have you been looking forward to the next episode of a Hulu show, watch that! Do you have a favorite podcast, tune in! Do you enjoy drawing? Perfect!

When you sleep well, anything you do before going to bed will become a cue for sleep and you'll have that relaxing bedtime routine people are talking about.

Looking forward to the hour before bed is an important step in this direction. Spending hours in a sensory deprivation chamber is not a sweet reward after a long day. Binging on that show you're just dying to catch the next episode of, now that's a different story!

Wait a minute... won't doing something fun wake me up and make me lose more sleep?

If that thought popped up in your head, then you have indeed identified a problem, and a big one too - your fear of losing sleep.

Every single person who has trouble sleeping is afraid of losing sleep. If they didn't they wouldn't have insomnia. Please know that every word in this book, including those about watching Hulu instead of avoiding screens, is here to help you teach your brain that it has nothing to fear. When you have no fear, you will sleep fantastic. This is inevitable and this is where you're going.

And remember, every time you do something at bedtime for the purpose of pleasure and not to avoid losing sleep, you are giving your brain a lesson in fearlessness.

HOW TO GET BACK TO SLEEP

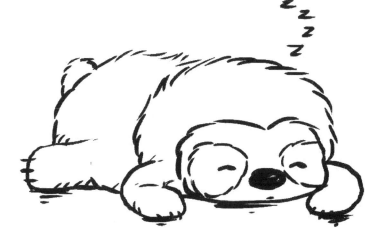

One of the most common questions someone with insomnia has is what to do when waking up at night. Or when going to bed and not falling asleep in a long time. You probably have this question too.

If you think about it, this is mostly (not always, noted!) a camouflaged way of asking how one can get back to sleep. Or even more bluntly put - what can I do to make myself fall asleep again? And at this point, you already know what trying to make yourself sleep is called and what happens when you do that.

Right again! It's a sleep effort and it produces sleeplessness.

Knowing this you already know the first of 5 key insights:

1. You can't force it

Hearing that you can't make yourself sleep may sound discouraging, unless you think of it as the complete opposite. Knowledge is power. You've just been empowered.

Knowing that you can accept things you can't change keeps you from falling into the rabbit hole of fighting reality. When you fight reality you lose. But only 100% of the time.

Also, keep in mind that acceptance is very different from resignation. Resigning means giving up, surrendering. Accepting means simply acknowledging reality. It is 76 degrees outside. My effective tax rate is 37%. It's not time to sleep right now.

When you accept that you're not ready for sleep, you can explore other options.

2. Resist the urge

When you wake up in the middle of the night, or you've been awake for what feels like an eternity after going to bed, you are going to want to know what time it is.

Or rather, your amygdala, your brain's safety system does. It wants to assess the damage so far and continue keeping a monitoring eye on the threat of losing more sleep.

Now ask yourself this question, how many times have you woken up as if you slept a long time, feeling wide awake, checked the time and felt a wave of relief. It's 2:37 am, fantastic! How many times have you gone on to feel so reassured and relaxed knowing that you've slept 1 hour and 37 minutes that you promptly fell back asleep.

Probably never. Or very rarely.

Knowing the time feels important. This is because your amygdala perceives sleeplessness as a threat that needs to be monitored. But it isn't.

In fact it is important that you don't know what time it is. This is another opportunity to teach your brain that it has nothing to be afraid of.

Resist the urge to check the time.

3. Take a mental journey

When you wake up or haven't fallen asleep in a long time (without knowing how many minutes, resist the urge!), think of something pleasant. If you feel comfortable in your warm bed and thinking of something pleasant comes easy to you - stay there and enjoy! You're likely to fall back asleep soon.

If you on the other hand find it difficult to think of something pleasant, if your thoughts revert back to your sleep, if you start getting frustrated then you need to shift focus. You can stay in bed as long as something like reading a book, listening to a podcast or watching TV grabs your attention.

Screens have no impact on insomnia, they're not a problem in themselves. However, it can be difficult to use a screen without getting to know the time.

If staying in bed and doing something enjoyable doesn't shift your attention, if you continue feeling frustrated, then leave the bed and do something you like doing elsewhere.

4. You can't trick yourself

You may wonder why there's so much emphasis here on doing something that you enjoy when you're not sleeping. Or at least something neutral like doing the dishes or some other chore that needs to get done.

Here's the thing - if you decide to pick up a really boring book or watch a show you've seen 200 times then what are you actually doing?

Yup, you got it. You're trying to make yourself sleep.

5. Have a playbook

Have you seen a football coach in action? Then you've seen someone who doesn't spend time deliberating what to do next. They already know. Because they have a playbook.

Having a playbook neutralizes a big sleep killer, wondering what to do if you wake up at night.

Be prepared. Know what show to watch or what book to read or whatever it is you want to do. And know this:

When you do all of the above and get to a point where you no longer fear having and early morning awakening, when you genuinely look forward to spending some time reading in that cozy corner you've prepared - you start sleeping all night long.

THE SLEEP HYGIENE TRAP

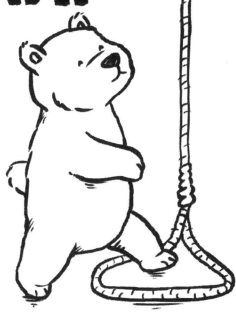

If there's one thing you most definitely have come across as you've had trouble sleeping, it is sleep hygiene. This term describes a laundry list of do's and don'ts that supposedly will help you sleep better.

Here are some common ones:

- » Go to bed and get out of bed the same time every day
- » Avoid screens and light an hour before you go to bed
- » Avoid caffeine close to bedtime
- » Make sure your bedroom is cool, 67-68 degrees for optimal sleep
- » Keep the noise level low
- » Avoid heavy/rich/spicy food close to bedtime

For some reason these recommendations have become an obligatory part of every article, story or blog post on sleep. This is odd because we've known for decades that sleep hygiene doesn't work.

Even worse - it creates a huge amount of sleep anxiety because of the implication that sleep is controllable and complicated!

There are only two things that determine how well we sleep...

...that's right, the gas and the brake!

The reason it is so important for you to know that sleep is simple, super simple, is that complexity and ambiguity creates anxiety.

A long list of do's and don'ts makes you believe that you have to get all of these things right, you have to check all the boxes, in order to sleep better. When you go on to have a sleepless night you feel you must be doing something wrong. You tweak and tinker and chase your tail in an endless cycle of self-experimentation and self-monitoring.

It's time to forget all about sleep hygiene, dial down the sleep anxiety and start catching some of those refreshing Zzzs!

Wait a minute...

...does what I eat and how active I am during the day and all those other things have absolutely no impact on my sleep?

Not entirely the case, but they're not the problem. It's your thinking that they are the problem that is the problem.

Confused? Hold tight, clarity is coming your way!

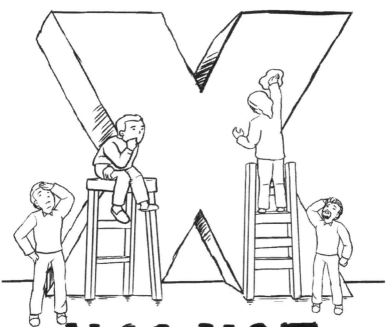

Let's get right to it - x is not the problem, you wondering if x is the problem is. It may not look like much, but this simple formula answers any question you have about what causes your troubles sleeping.

And here's why.:

A million and a half things can disrupt your sleep. Bed bugs, smelly socks, hot flashes, your neighbors cat, your hormone levels, the linings of your pillow, a medication you're taking, you name it. There's simply no end to any and all of the things that can have some impact on how you sleep.

But only one thing can cause you to struggle with sleep night after night, week after week, year after year - your thoughts and habits.

It's as simple as that.

Think about that friend of yours who sleeps really well. Ask her how she does that and you'll just get a blank stare. Huh, dunno? I just sleep…

This doesn't mean that her sleep is not affected at all by medications or loud noises, but the impact is so small that she doesn't even notice it or think about it.

Is it possible that the extra spicy veggie korma you had made you sleep 3 minutes less. Sure. Could your Propranolol make you sleep 4 minutes more. That's possible. Could your hot flashes wake you up drenched in sweat so you sleep 25 minutes less. Absolutely.

Could any of the above explain why it takes you hours to fall asleep or why you get your best sleep at 5 am or why nothing works or why you can't sleep in general? Absolutely not.

When that thought pops up in your brain, when you wonder if this thing or that is the reason you're not sleeping well, plug it into this sentence - x is not the problem, me wondering if x is the problem is.

Whatever it is, plug it in and you'll soon stop wondering why you're not sleeping. When you stop wondering, you become less preoccupied, less anxious and guess what, sleep better!

FOUR STAGES OF RECOVERY

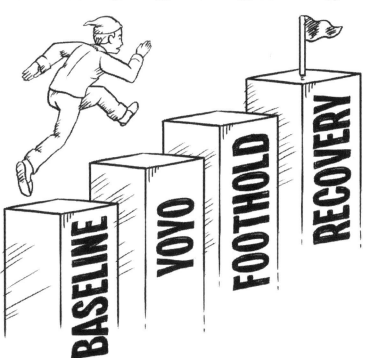

Starting any journey, you naturally wonder when you will reach your destination. When will we land? When will I have enough savings to retire? When is my burrito going to be done? No matter what path you're on, the exact time until that final step is often uncertain. That is true for getting past insomnia as well. But that doesn't mean you can't see where on the road map you are.

There are four stages when you Set it & Forget it - Baseline, Yo-Yo, Foothold and Recovery. Let's explore them to give you a sense of where you are and what to expect.

Baseline

This is the stage you're in before you start using Set it & Forget it. It may have lasted weeks, months, years or even decades. In the baseline stage your sleep confidence is low, you're worried about sleep, there is little predictability and you have predominantly nights of little sleep.

Yo-yo

The yo-yo stage starts as soon as you start learning about insomnia and spending less time in bed. It typically lasts 2-4 weeks. This said, some get past it even faster than 2 weeks and for others it may take more than 4. Don't be discouraged if you're in the latter group - you will get there as long as you keep going.

In the yo-yo stage sleep still feels unpredictable, you have predominantly nights of little sleep and your sleep confidence is still low - but, there are positive signs. And that's a big deal.

You may have had a few nights where you fell asleep a little faster than usual or you fell back asleep when you wouldn't have done that in the past.

Also, as you're understanding why you have trouble sleeping, as you see that this is a common problem and nothing is wrong with you - you start worrying less. And that's also a big deal. Because after worrying decreases, sleep starts to come easier.

What is really important in the yo-yo stage is to hold on to any little positive sign. Focus on any hint of improvement. Tell a friend. Write it down. Affirming that there are hopeful indicators becomes stepping stones. Stepping stones that allow you to move forward faster and with increasing confidence.

Foothold

The foothold stage comes after the yo-yo stage and usually lasts 3-5 weeks. This is a stage of gradual improvement. Worrying about sleep decreases. You start seeing that you can sleep, sleep confidence increases. There are still nights of little sleep but mostly you sleep well and sleep seems more predictable.

Most importantly - once you reach the foothold stage, there's no turning back. You are on a path to recovery and you can now see the light at the end of the tunnel. This is why during the previous yo-yo stage it is crucial that you keep moving forward no matter how stressful and chaotic it can seem.

Recovery

This final stage lasts indefinitely. You are not worried about sleep. Even if you have nights of little sleep, you know that this is normal and you don't react to them. Your sleep confidence is good. You feel that sleep is predictable and you no longer keep track of how much you sleep.

Most importantly, and the reason it lasts a lifetime, you've understood that your thoughts and habits were the reasons you had trouble sleeping. You easily resist any urge to figure out why you have a stretch of little sleep or an occasional sleepless night.

As you can see, recovery really all hinges upon not giving up during the yo-yo stage. Use this road map to give you a boost of motivation when you need to see the light at the end of the tunnel.

ARE YOU SLEEPY OR TIRED?

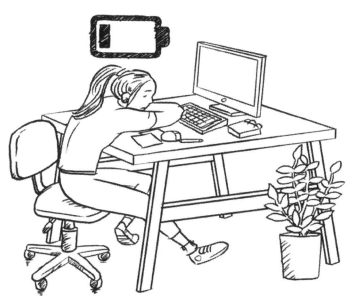

Listening to your body is a common tip that makes a lot of sense. However, sometimes the problem isn't that we aren't listening but that we misinterpret what our bodies are trying to tell us. This is very common with insomnia and can make it really difficult to get good and predictable sleep. Let's make sure you are tuned in to your body's signals and dodge this speed bump.

Being tired is a feeling of lack of energy. It's feeling exhausted or fatigued. Sometimes it is mostly a physical sensation, your body feels drained. Other times it is more of a mental fatigue whereby you feel foggy and have a hard time concentrating or remembering things.

Being sleepy on the other hand is when your eyelids feel heavy and sleeping feels irresistible. You know you could easily drift off. You nod off and have to read paragraphs multiple times.

When you feel tired, your body is telling you that you either need to rest or do the opposite, become more active and get your blood pumping.

When you feel sleepy your body is signaling that it wants you to sleep. Sometimes sleepiness occurs at the right time and you should go to bed. Other times you have to disregard the message and stay up until an appropriate time to sleep.

A common problem that happens when you're mixing up fatigue and sleepiness is that you think you should sleep when you're in fact not sleepy. You feel drained and exhausted and go to bed. However, as you weren't actually sleepy you simply end up tossing and turning which makes you even more tired. Or you may have some superficial brief sleep that is no more refreshing.

Make sure you don't go to bed unless you're sleepy. It can take some time to retrain yourself to recognize your body's cues. Keep at it and you will soon know the signals and the right response. You will know when it is time to hit the gym, the couch or the bed and feel much better!

THE 17 HOUR RULE

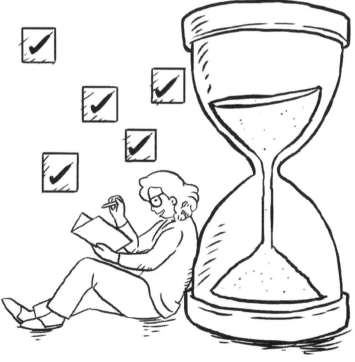

One of the most common pieces of unhelpful advice you've most likely heard many times is to go to bed at the same time every night. In addition to this one, there's a host of related tips that all make you believe that bedtime is really important. These are things like lists of what to do and not to do before going to bed and tips about how to create a bedtime ritual. We've covered that.

In reality, it's in the opposite part of the day/night cycle where sleep is created. To see why this is the case, let's look at the 17 hour rule.

Imagine someone who sleeps 7 hours per night, let's call her Emma. Subtract her 7 hours of sleep from the 24 hours in a day/night and you get 17. This, 17, is the number of hours of wakefulness she needs to produce 7 hours of sleep.

Let's repeat that, Emma needs 17 hours of wakefulness to produce 7 hours of sleep.

It may not sound earth shaking, but this insight is super important. You'll see why in a second.

Imagine Emma getting up at 7 am. When will she be ready to sleep?

That's right, around midnight. 17 hours after 7 am. Because it takes 17 hours of wakefulness to get her to a place where she is ready to sleep.

Now imagine that she had a very restless night. She only slept a few hours and instead of getting up at her usual 7 am, she decides to sleep in to make up for lost sleep. She gets some sleep from 7 am until 9:30 am after which she gets up.

Now when will she be ready to sleep?

Yup exactly, at 2:30 am.

This seems pretty obvious when you understand sleep physiology. But for Emma who's never heard of the 17 hours rule it seems strange that she can't fall asleep when she usually goes to bed at midnight.

Perhaps the most important thing to learn from this rule is that mornings are what matter. You can tweak and tinker all you want with bedtime, but that's not going to change whether you're ready to sleep or not. Sleep is a consequence of wakefulness. When sleep happens is a consequence of when wakefulness happens.

Another important learning point is that sleeping in after a night of getting little sleep is very disruptive to your sleep patterns. This is why it's good to get up about the same time every morning when you have trouble sleeping.

By the way, if you need 6 hours of sleep, then it's the 18 hour rule for you. If you need 8 then you should pay attention to the 16 hour rule.

Whatever rule applies to you, use your new knowledge to set the stage for solid sleep starting today.

Correction, tomorrow morning.

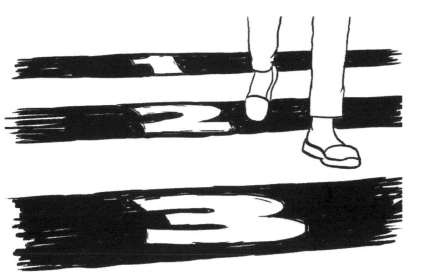

THE THREE STEPS

The roadmap towards sleeping well has four stages as we've seen. There's another important thing to know about the journey you're on. From a less detailed, big picture perspective there are three big steps - worrying less, sleeping better and feeling less tired. Here's why this is good to know.

One of the most common things you will hear someone say after a week or two of using Set it & Forget it is that they're starting to feel less worried, but sleep no better. Mostly this is brought up as a concern. I'm starting to understand and I'm not as anxious, so why isn't sleep improving yet?

As your goal is to sleep and feel better, worrying less doesn't seem like something to celebrate. In reality, when you worry less, you've taken a big leap forward.

It takes time for sleep patterns to change. Particularly if you've had trouble sleeping for years, or even decades. Simply starting to feel that insomnia is less of a mystery and understanding why you've had difficulties is a big step. And the next one, better sleep, is soon to follow.

Just to be super clear, the first step is understanding and worrying less, and the second step is better sleep.

What you also often hear people say is that they're still tired even though they sleep better. Again, this is often presented as a concern - my sleep has improved so why am I not more rested?

This is another very encouraging thing to hear. The hyperarousal is now low enough that it allows good sleep but, interestingly this can actually produce more fatigue. Or rather, unmask it.

When insomnia is active, your brain is in flight of fight mode. Adrenaline is pumping and your central nervous system is in high gear. All this hyperarousal can keep you from noticing how tiring it is to be constantly on guard. You literally don't feel how exhausted you are.

Once the hyperarousal lifts, you start sleeping better but you also start feeling the full unmasked fatigue resulting from the high gear you've been in. The fatigue is actually a positive sign, a sign that the struggle is over.

When you've slept better for a while, you'll stop feeling tired.

And you've taken that third and last step.

So what have we learned here?

If you worry less but still don't sleep more, or if you sleep better but still feel fatigued - just keep going. Good things are coming your way.

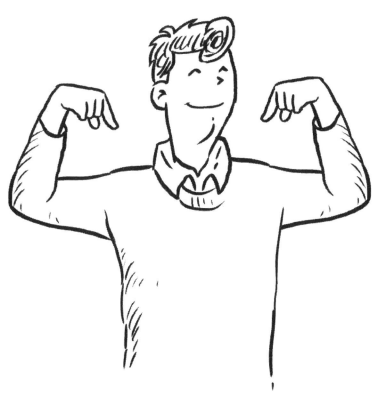

If you take medications to sleep and/or want to stop doing that, this chapter is for you. We will start with the problem, which may be a different one than you expect, and then move on to the solution.

Imagine someone starting to have trouble sleeping, let's call her Alexa. She's slept well until a stressful move to a new state. She goes through a bunch of supplements and sleep hygiene tips without getting any better and soon starts believing something is wrong with her.

After several sleepless months she decides it is time to see her doctor. The doctor tells her she has insomnia and prescribes some Ambien.

This is a critical moment.

Two things have happened that are very problematic.

Firstly, Alexa's fears have been confirmed, there is something wrong with her. She has a condition called insomnia.

Secondly, the implied message when given a prescription is that she cannot sleep on her own.

What happens next is just as critical.

Either Alexa takes her Ambien and sleeps no better. Now she really feels something is wrong with her. Not even prescription strength medications can make her sleep. Or, she takes her Ambien and she finally sleeps. This is the worst case scenario. Because the fact that she slept after taking medication confirms what the doctor said - something is wrong inside her and she cannot sleep on her own.

Alexa's already shaky sleep confidence now starts to completely erode.

You know something Alexa didn't. Only your sleep drive can produce sleep. Medications cannot.

So why, you may wonder, is it that Alexa slept after taking Ambien in the second scenario?

Sleep happens when there's enough gas and little braking going on. Medications cannot produce a solid sleep drive, but they can temporarily easy up on the gas. Either by a direct placebo effect, Alexa believes it will help and therefore she's less hyperaroused. Or an indirect placebo effect, Alexa becomes sedated and unable to create thoughts that are complex enough to make her hyperaroused.

It may seem like splitting hairs to go to this length to show that medications don't make you sleep. But it's not. It's super important. Because when you believe anything except yourself is making you sleep, your confidence suffers. And without sleep confidence, you will continue having trouble sleeping.

Going back to Alexa, you may wonder if it's really all that bad if she takes Ambien and sleeps well?

Here's the thing, there's no evidence that taking sleep medication causes any serious health problems. It's likely that they increase falls among the elderly and they surely can make you feel groggy and hungover. But that's not the big problem for most. Rather it is that they make you very vulnerable.

Let's say Alexa takes Ambien for a few months and sleeps better. At this point, she's completely habituated to the sedating effect of the medication and the effect of the sleeping pill is 100% confidence boosting, aka placebo.

Now something changes. Her landlord increases the rent or she breaks up with her boyfriend or her pet hamster dies and suddenly, Ambien stops working. Or so it seems. In reality, what happens is just like when a magician has you believing there's a coin in his hand until he suddenly reveals an empty palm. The coin wasn't there in the first place, but the reveal is no less dramatic. Alexa's confidence was boosted by a medication but with increased stress, that boost was insufficient and she has insomnia again.

And now she's really in a bind. She feels like her insomnia has taken a life of its own. It has changed. Nothing can control it. She goes back to her doctor who increases the prescription strength and a new round of confidence destruction starts.

Now to more positive territory - sleep confidence can be rebuilt!

Alexa can go on to sleep amazingly well as long as she does the thought work and habit change that you're doing. And here's how to do that if you're taking medication.

Firstly it is super important to make any medication you take a non factor. It has to become something you know has no influence over how well you sleep. There are two ways of doing that. Either you take the medication the same time, same dosage every single night like a robot or you don't take it at all. In both scenarios, you will know that whether you had a great night or one of little sleep had nothing to do with the medication.

In other words, taking sleep aids only when needed is to be avoided. This is very important because if you decide to wait and see, then you will start self monitoring. You will be querying yourself to see if you should take it or not. You will be wondering if you should maybe take half. You'll ask yourself how much longer you should wait. This builds a ton of anxiety that in no way helps you sleep. Also, if you finally cave in after 4 hours and take that pill, you have just trained your brain that sleeplessness is dangerous and that you can't sleep by yourself.

Now how about if you want to stop taking medication, how should you do that?

The most important thing here is that you don't consider it an experiment, if you do, you'll never be successful.

If you set out to see how many nights you can go without taking a sleep aid, then your preoccupation and anxiety levels will mount day by day, with less and less sleep at night. You keep soldiering on, determined not to give up, but after a stretch of nearly completely sleepless nights you finally can't do it anymore and go back on your medication.

What caused you to have such strong rebound insomnia had nothing to do with the absence of a chemical in your brain, rather it was the fact that you approached coming off as an experiment.

Coming off a sleep aid has to be a decision. You decide on which date you stop and never look back. If you give yourself any opportunity to go back on the sleep aid, then it's an experiment. If you never look back, then you will be successful.

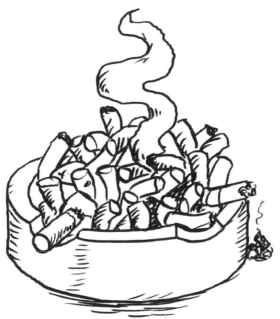

ASHTRAYS ARE iNNOCENT

Did you know that ashtrays are associated with COPD? If not, do know that there is a strong link between the two. There is even a dose-response relationship:

The more ash trays someone has, the more likely they are to have COPD.

Does this mean that ash trays cause COPD? That they are the reason people with ashtrays have more lung problems?

That has never been proven. In fact it is believed that it is smoking cigarettes that is the culprit and not those ashtrays.

Now what does this have to do with sleep? Quite a bit it turns out.

Sleep is like the ash trays in this example. Many health issues have been associated with sleep problems, but a causal relationship has never been found. And here are two things that's really important to know - it is impossible to prove that short sleep causes health problems and long sleep is much more strongly linked to such problems.

Let's look first at the feasibility of proving that short sleep causes for example Alzheimer's disease. To prove that one thing causes another you will need a randomized study with two imposed conditions. You need thousands of people and you need to make half of them sleep deprived as you make sure the other half sleeps a lot. After decades of maintaining both groups of short and long sleepers respectively, you could look at whether Alzheimer's happened more in the sleep deprived or non sleep deprived group.

Needless to say - a study like this will never happen. Therefore it is not possible to prove that short sleep causes any disease or health issue.

This is important for you to know because whenever you see a headline trying to make you believe that some researcher has found that short sleep causes this or that health issue, that's not true. They've just found an association.

They've just asked a bunch of people how much they sleep and then checked if the answer could be correlated to whether they have diabetes or heart disease or whatever other health problem they were looking at.

And guess what studies like these always show? People who estimate sleeping more than 7 hours and less than 6 hours have more health issues. In fact sleeping 8 hours is just as "dangerous" as sleeping 4.5 hours. This fact is conveniently overlooked in a world where attention is the currency of success. Who would read an article that says that sleeping 8 hours is linked to diabetes?

Researchers, non profits, bloggers, traditional media and mattress salespeople all need your attention to generate grants, advertising revenue and sales. This is why you never hear that the link between health issues and sleep is much stronger for long than for short sleep.

But wait a minute you may say. Why is there a link to begin with?

This is because health issues can affect how much you estimate sleeping in both directions. Having arthritis and pain can disrupt your sleep and lower your estimated sleep time. Heart failure can make you tired, spend more time in bed and increase the amount of time you feel that you sleep.

When you think about it, wouldn't you be more surprised if health issues had no impact on sleep whatsoever?

There's no mystery as for why there's a link between sleep and health. Health issues almost always cause sleep problems. But the opposite has never been proven. In fact it cannot be proven as we have seen above.

But how about a cohort study?

How about if you just ask people if they have trouble sleeping or not and then check whether this predicts health outcomes.

This has been done many times. And the results are very consistent.

When you ask people whether they have trouble sleeping or not (as opposed to asking people to estimate how much they sleep) and then look at outcomes years later, you find that people who reported having insomnia and those who didn't have the exact same life expectancy.

Knowing that short sleep or insomnia, despite what you hear, never have been shown to cause any health issues is important.

Because as you know, worrying less is the first step towards sleeping amazing!

FORGET iT

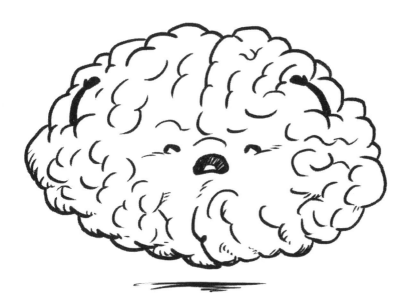

One of the most common things that keep people from sleeping well, or sleeping at all, is anxiety. Sometimes this is general anxiety that spills over onto sleep. Sometimes the source of the anxiety is strictly that worry of whether or not you will sleep, how much you will sleep and what will happen if you don't.

If you have mostly sleep anxiety, then the good news is that it's not too difficult to get past. Set it & Forget it works great for sleep anxiety. This is because the cure for sleep anxiety is sleeping well. Set it & Forget it takes you there.

If you have more general anxiety, or want to speed up the process of reducing sleep anxiety, then you should try focused journaling.

As you know, with anxiety comes the constant bombardment of thoughts produced by your brain. Without an outlet, it is up to you to react and respond to all the whims of an overactive mind. If all this activity on the other hand can be directed towards a designated time frame, the bombardment will cease.

Here's what to do:

In the early afternoon, set off 5-10 minutes and grab a pen and paper. During these minutes, try to get every single worry you can retrieve from your mind written down. The more material you find, the more stressors and worries you identify, the better.

Don't expect anything to change in the first few days. But if you keep going, just like with any exercise, you will start seeing results. When your brain has an outlet, it will bother you less and give you more peace of mind to spend on things you enjoy.

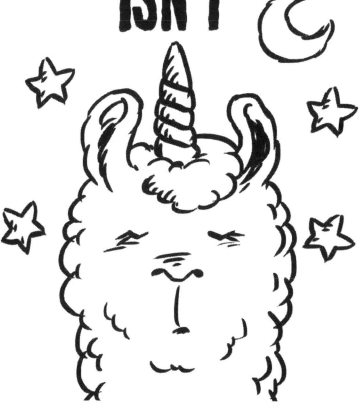

Many with trouble sleeping feel that their situation is different from that of others with insomnia. From the perspective of a coach, it is notable how client after client describes the exact same problems yet all believe they're going through something unusual and unique.

It's not hard to see why this happens. We shall explore this in a second because it is very important. And here's why: Believing that your insomnia is unique takes you down a path of looking for a unique underlying reason and unique treatment. A journey that only leads to more confusion and frustration. Believing that your insomnia is ordinary on the other hand, leads you to see how the approach described here, that works for so many others, will also work for you.

No matter how hard you're being pulled down the rabbit hole into the land of Oz where things are bizarre and fantastic, stay in Kansas.

Let's start at the very beginning - someone going through a series of sleepless nights.

From the inside perspective, not sleeping for a stretch of time can seem very strange. Sleeping being something very natural, like eating or thinking, it can seem bizarre that it just isn't happening.

But as mentioned, this is just the beginning.

Next, having become a bit worried and perplexed, you want to do something about the fact that sleep isn't happening. Surely taking some melatonin and keeping the bedroom dark should take care of it.

When nothing changes, perplexed becomes confused. When even more efforts make no difference, confused becomes clueless. And the insomnia at this point starts seeming strange and unique. You feel you've got an usual case because it didn't respond to anything or because of other circumstances including:

- » You have no trouble falling asleep, just staying asleep
- » You don't feel sleepy during the day
- » You suddenly feel awake or jerk just as you're about to sleep
- » You have no trouble staying asleep, just falling asleep

» You sleep the best just as the sun rises

» You've had trouble sleeping all your life

» The type of sleep itself is strange, you have vivid dreams all the time a you're never fully asleep

» People tell you you sleep but you don't feel like you sleep at all

Here's the thing, we are all unique human beings. Your experiences are unique and many circumstances surrounding your troubles sleeping are unique - but your insomnia isn't.

Either there's too little gas or too much braking going on. Anything bizarre happening, hyperarousal is the culprit.

That's it.

Although it may not seem like it, nothing else matters when it comes to insomnia.

There are many reasons why you may feel that your troubles sleeping are different, strange and unique. They're not. Neither is the belief that your troubles are different, strange or unique. It is a very common and ordinary belief.

This is not to belittle what you're going through. Saying that your insomnia is not unique is not saying that it hasn't had a big impact on your life. But the belief that you have a different kind of insomnia will keep you in a sleepless loop.

Believing on the other hand that you are a unique and special person, but that your insomnia is ordinary, everyday, uninteresting, garden variety insomnia will make you see how you, just like anyone else with regular insomnia, will sleep well with a method like Set it & Forget it!

CORE SLEEP

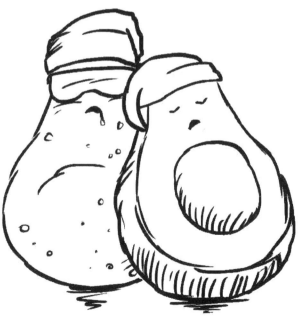

Have you ever wondered how it is that you can go for weeks on almost no sleep? Perhaps you've felt like you're muddling through, feeling tired and foggy.

Perhaps on the contrary you've found it puzzling that you have so much energy despite sleeping so little.

There's more than one reason the above happens, it could be any combination of too little gas, too much brake or both, but a key to demystifying what you're experiencing lies in the concept of core sleep.

We all need a certain amount of sleep to feel rested and refreshed. However, in times of stress or excitement (or any other form of hyperarousal) sleep need is decreased. As you know, this is a normal reaction. Sleeping less and waking up more often is a perfect survival mechanism when we are under threat. The question becomes: How little can we sleep?

It turns out that this number is four hours.

Or so we believe. There aren't any randomized studies but looking at data models you find the following:

If someone sleeps about four hours per night they can remain awake and somehow get through the remaining 20 hours for weeks. Getting less than four hours per night on the other hand leads to crashes. The system will shut down periodically to reboot and resume operations.

So why is this important to know?

Here's the thing - if you spend seven hours in bed and sleep four, but those four hours of sleep are fragmented and superficial, it may feel like you only slept 2 hours. As we can sustain operational ability on four hours of sleep, it can seem like you're sleeping almost nothing at all and still stay awake during the day. It may feel like you're barely keeping it together, or if you're a very high energy person, you may still have reserves and feel strangely alert.

What is happening in either case is that you are living on core sleep. The minimum amount your body/brain can keep things running on.

Don't get me wrong, living on core sleep is not where you want to be, it's not something you should resign to. It certainly shouldn't be your goal! But understanding how you can go for weeks on what feels like almost no sleep is important for your insomnia to seem less bizarre and unusual.

What to do?
Set it & Forget it! As your hyperarousal comes down you will sleep more, perceive sleeping more and leave core sleep behind.

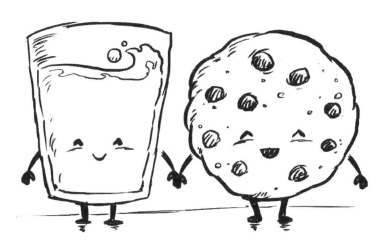

HOLD ON
TO THAT
COOKiE

One of the most common questions people with trouble sleeping have is whether one should stop drinking coffee completely or limit intake after a certain hour. It's the perfect example of giving a mouse a cookie. If you're not familiar with that children's book, here's a synopsis:

A mouse asks a boy for a cookie. Having finished the cookie, the mouse asks for some milk. After that it needs a mirror to see if it got a milk moustache, then scissors to trim its whiskers. This continues until it finally asks for some more milk - and a cookie to go with it.

The key insight here is that by giving the mouse more and more of what it asks for, the boy is becoming more and more manipulated and powerless. The more the mouse gets, the more it wants in a never ending cycle of failed appeasement.

Insomnia works just the same. Your amygdala has identified sleeplessness as a threat and is asking you to give up things in an effort to neutralize the threat. When your amygdala feels no less threatened, it asks you to give something else up.

As you can see, the more things you give up the bigger of a problem insomnia becomes. And it will stop at nothing. It can literally become an obsession that consumes your night and day.

This is why you have to hold on to every cookie you have. Don't give up coffee. Don't give up a trip you've looked forward to. Don't give up that late night party.

Give the cookie to someone who needs a sweet reward - yourself.

THE RABBIT HOLES OF INSOMNIA

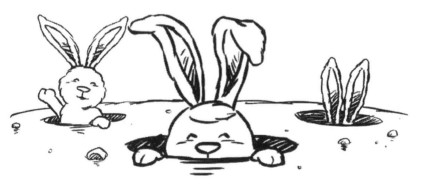

Take a look at this definition of going down the rabbit hole while imagining yourself or someone else having trouble sleeping:

"To enter into a situation or begin a process or journey that is particularly strange, problematic, difficult, complex, or chaotic, especially one that becomes increasingly so as it develops or unfolds."

Anyone familiar with insomnia easily recognizes this description as being spot on. Particularly the entanglement, the getting increasingly worse as the trip continues part.

Here's the thing - one can look at developing insomnia as one trip down the rabbit hole, or many.

Imagine a universe where there are multiple insomnia rabbit holes, each producing sleeplessness albeit by different means. Let's explore these rabbit holes so you know where not to go.

Sleep optimization - You're sleeping ok but don't feel refreshed during the day. You feel tired and don't know why. You decide that perhaps you're not getting good sleep quality and that it's time to do something about this. You try supplements, perhaps some CBD oil but feel not better. In fact, you're surprised nothing is making a difference. As you try more things to get better sleep quality, you notice that you're sleeping less and less and need to double down on your efforts. You've gone down the sleep optimization rabbit hole.

Wellness improvement - You're an active person that likes to be in good shape. Not only physical but mental wellness is important to you. You exercise and do yoga but haven't paid much attention to sleep. You decide to make now the time to improve your sleep and purchase some essential oils and use a fitbit to keep track of how you're doing. You realize you're only getting 30 minutes of deep sleep per night and this is with the essential oils. You decide to meditate more. The tracker results don't budge. You have to do more. You've gone down the wellness improvement rabbit hole.

Sleep envy - You've never slept that much or that great, but on the other hand sleep hasn't been a problem for you. You note however that your partner sleeps a solid 8 hours every night. You would like that too. You start going to bed earlier but nothing changes. You start using a sleep mask and ear plugs but now actually sleep less. You start looking for ways to sleep more. You've gone down the sleep envy rabbit hole.

Health anxiety - You've not had any problems with sleep but read an article saying it's important to get between 7-9 hours to minimize the risk of having a stroke. You read up on sleep hygiene and decide to go to bed and get up the same time every night but still only get 6 hours of sleep. You stop drinking coffee but things don't get any better. You stop watching TV in the evening and still stay well short of the recommended amount, you need to do more. You've gone down the health anxiety rabbit hole.

Avoiding these rabbit holes is the key to not having insomnia. If you've gone down one on the other hand, you can use the above insights to pull yourself up.

And to do that, it's important to note what they all have in common -attention. Trying to sleep more, tracking how many hours you sleep, focusing on sleep are all variations of giving sleep attention. Without attention, insomnia fades away.

So climb up your rabbit hole by spending less time in bed and no time at all trying to figure out why you're not sleeping more or what you can do to get more sleep.

This is the path up any rabbit hole and back to a place of sleeping well.

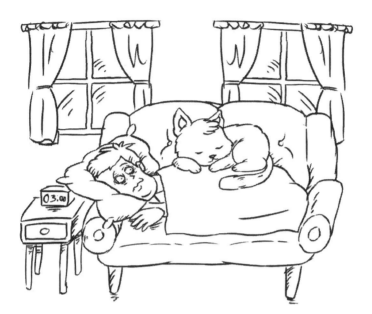

BLAME IT ON HYPERAROUSAL

Even if you've never heard of it or used the word, you have felt it. Defined as "an abnormal state of increased responsiveness to stimuli that is marked by various physiological and psychological symptoms" hyperarousal comes in many shapes and forms.

Remember that time you were lying awake in bed as a child, hardly able to wait to open presents the next day? That's an example of a time when you were hyperaroused, this time in the shape of excitement.

That other time, when the thought of a presentation gave you palpitations, hyperarousal came in the shape of anxiety.

Not only are there different causes for hyperarousal, but different intensity levels. From the slightest awareness of being on edge to a full blown panic attack.

Here's the thing - hyperarousal is always the culprit. At least when it comes to insomnia.

Most with trouble sleeping have no problem whatsoever recognizing that worry or anxiety is why they can't sleep. Either the anxiety is about sleep itself or general anxiety spills over into sleep. However, there are other things that often happen where the reason is not as obvious:

Twitches. A weird tension. A sudden awareness of falling asleep that jolts you awake. A surge of energy. Recurring leg or body jerks when you were just drifting off to sleep. These are all caused by hyperarousal.

Racing thoughts. Palpitations. Feeling weirdly awake during the day even after only having slept 2 hours. Being in a constant state of half-wakefulness at night. Extremely vivid dreams. Feeling like you haven't slept at all for days. Having to pee all the time. Yup, hyperarousal again.

Nothing is going on. You're not worried about anything and somehow you're only sleeping a few hours per night. This is the most subtle form, ninja style hyperarousal.

So what to do if you have hyperarousal?

Actually, what not to do is an even better place to start. And that is because doing anything with the direct intent of reducing hyperarousal will backfire.

If you decide to start meditating, well then you're going to be self-monitoring, checking how the meditation is working, giving hyperarousal more attention which makes it stronger.

If you start jogging more, you'll be wondering how many more miles you have to run before you feel less anxious, making you more anxious.

As much as you want to focus on getting rid of the hyperarousal, you have to go in the opposite direction.

You have to find things that are inherently enjoyable. Things you do simply for pleasure. If it involves other people, even better. That will distract you even more from the hyperarousal that's been bothering you.

When hyperarousal is no more, all those weird sleep related things that were keeping you awake will stop happening. Simply knowing what hyperarousal is, demystifying what has seemed strange, is a great step in the right direction.

TURNING LEMONS INTO LEMONADE

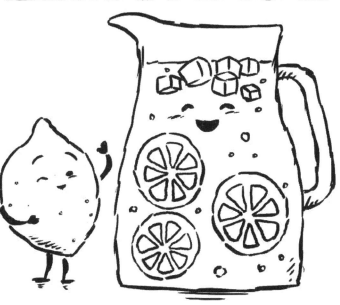

Nobody wants a sleepless night, whether you have trouble sleeping or not. It is a lemon. This said, there are many ways to look at a night where you didn't get a wink from a different perspective. A perspective from which you see how these are opportunities to take big steps towards amazing sleep.

Let's start with the most straight forward insight, wakefulness produces sleep so with more wakefulness your chances of sleeping well will increase.

As you know the one thing that can make a human sleep is your sleep drive. This is your body's need for sleep, the gas in our sleep system. If you hardly sleep at all for an entire night, then your sleep drive the following night will be much stronger and solid sleep more likely. The trick is not giving in to the temptation of catching up in the morning or sleeping during the day. You'll need all that gas later.

Now here's a perhaps even more important opportunity that comes from being awake all night - reducing the fear of sleep loss.

The fear of losing sleep almost always drives your insomnia. It creates anxiety that makes it hard to sleep. It creates unhelpful habits like trying to get sleep whenever you can by spending more time in bed. Now what if you could prove to yourself that even after not having slept at all, you can go through your day without any catastrophic event?

This is not easy by any means, not sleeping in itself plus the frustration with not sleeping can be exhausting. That is why this is the time to find those reserves. This is the time to mobilize every untapped energy resource you have and have a good day. Treat yourself! Go to the spa. Enjoy a delicious dessert.

This is super important because if you go on to have an ok day, or better yet a good one, then you may completely lose the fear of having a sleepless night. If you can get to a place where you don't mind having a sleepless night because you get to enjoy something you otherwise can't, you've taken a big step towards not having those nights.

Another way you can think about this is recalling that time you decided to pull an all nighter. You decided to study or you were having a great time with friends. You were literally awake the entire night and then had to go to work or school the next day. You probably felt tired, but guess what, you did fine. And you didn't obsess over the fact that you were awake all night, that was the whole idea!

There's nothing different between being up all night because you decided to do that or because of hyperarousal - except your thoughts around it. If you can change your thoughts and think of a sleepless night as pulling an all nighter, something you can do and still do fine the following day, you're at serious risk of never having a sleepless night again.

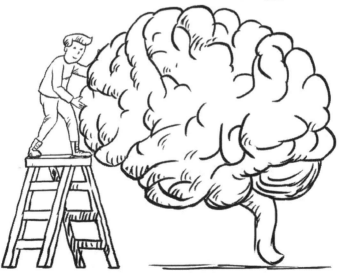

Some of the most common questions people with trouble sleeping have is whether it is true that insomnia can cause problems with your immune system or whether sleeplessness can cause psychosis. Often these questions come from articles you've read that are based on research studies.

It's tempting to review the original research paper to try to find out how reliable they are. Or ask an expert for their opinion. In other words, to get as close to the truth as possible.

As you know, this behavior is a form of threat monitoring - trying to get a grip of one's opponent to stay clear of harm. A great strategy for physical threats but not for perceived threats. A variety of threat monitoring that is also very problematic when it comes to perceived threats is truth finding. And here's why:

Looking for the truth when the truth cannot be established leaves you more frustrated, anxious and confused than before you started looking.

If we use the question of sleep and the immune system as an example, the only way to really know whether insomnia causes infections would be to take thousands of people and randomize them to an insomnia and a no insomnia condition and then check in which group you had more colds or pneumonia.

This is just not possible for several reasons, one being that there is no way to make someone have insomnia.

In other words, it is impossible to prove that insomnia causes any health issues, the truth cannot be established.

This said, the process of looking for the truth can make you feel like you're finding bread crumbs. You may feel like you're getting closer to the core of the matter which in its turn creates a belief that you should continue looking. You feel like you're making progress and that the act of truth finding is important.

In reality, you're just giving insomnia more attention which will make it more difficult for you to get to a place of good sleep.

Here's the thing, don't choose to believe something based on whether it is true or not. Consider truth unavailable. Instead, choose a belief that serves you well or, even better, decide not to even bother with choosing a belief.

Think of it as those existential questions we grapple with in our youth. It sometimes feels like you're getting closer to the answers when you talk to people and read books. But ultimately you learn to accept that there are no answers to be found and abandon the search.

It's good for you to believe that insomnia does nothing to your immune system. You can choose that belief. Or you can abandon any attempt at figuring out what insomnia does or doesn't do.

If you can, go for the latter, because when you give insomnia no attention, amazing sleep happens. If you go for the former, well that's fantastic as well. Because good things will come your way when you choose a good truth.

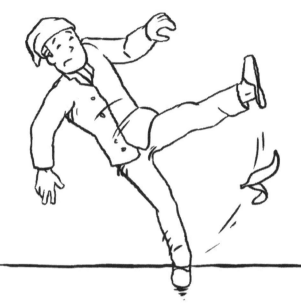

3 REASONS A SETBACK IS A GOOD THING

If you've started to Set it & Forget it and and started sleeping better only to have a stretch of little sleep - don't panic, something good is happening to you! Let's take a look at why this is a real opportunity and how you can take several steps forward after having taken one backwards.

Before we start though, a few words on what a setback is. Most people think of insomnia as having a life of its own. An entity that you can push down to the basement. But sometimes, if you're unlucky, it comes back. The problem with this belief is that it makes you feel disempowered. You're pushed into a defensive position where you can simply react to whatever insomnia is deciding to do.

This is a myth.

Reality is that insomnia is simply a product of your thoughts and habits.

When you sleep little after having slept better for some time, this simply means that you again have started thinking of sleeplessness as a threat. Insomnia does not have a life of its own, it only exists when your threat monitoring system decides that it exists.

This should make you feel empowered. You have complete control over what happens going forward and guess what. You've already done great work and your brain started looking at sleeplessness as less of a threat. You can do it again. And understanding these following three reasons a setback is a good thing can help you never have one again.

Firstly, you're in a place from which you can have a setback.

As humans we are naturally inclined to look at negatives. If our spouse didn't turn on the dishwasher for the second day in a row, that's an issue. But if they did, we don't celebrate, they're just doing what they're supposed to be doing. We always look for problems to fix, things to improve.

That's good! This is why we're doing so well as a species. However, sometimes focusing on the problem keeps us from seeing and celebrating our successes.

When someone has started sleeping better and then has a stretch of nights with little sleep, the news is that they started sleeping better! That's the part that is fantastic and fabulous and wonderful!

You have made so much progress that not sleeping feels like a step backwards. That is nothing short of amazing!
The first reason a setback is a good thing is that you've established a new baseline from which you can have a setback. It is super important to really obsess about the progress that you've made as this will grow your sleep confidence.

Secondly, it is in challenging times that you have the most opportunity.

Getting past insomnia is all about growing sleep confidence. When you're gradually getting better sleep over a course of a few weeks, you're starting to see that you CAN sleep and that there's nothing wrong with you. That's great of course. But if you've had trouble sleeping and put in a lot of effort trying to sleep for months or years, this slow and steady progress is not the most effective way of growing your sleep confidence.

When you have a setback on the other hand, when you're down to sleeping a few hours per night, you have potential for rapid growth. The trick though is to resist the urge to tinker.

If you go back to sleeping little and start trying to do

things to get back on track, you're spoiling your opportunity. Because if you change how much time you spend in bed or take a medication or do anything else that results in you sleeping more, you have missed a chance to see that you would have bounced back even if you had done nothing.

If you have a setback and you don't change a thing, if you just keep doing exactly what you were doing when you were sleeping better, that's when the magic happens. When you start sleeping better again, you have seen that you get back on track by doing nothing at all. You have seen that nothing but your own innate ability to sleep is needed to come back from a period of little sleep.

A comeback like that grows your confidence more than anything else.

Thirdly, you have a chance to find that you can have a great day even after sleeping little.

As with all anxiety, sleep anxiety is driven by fear of the unknown. And when you sleep little, those fears grow. What if I can't drive tomorrow? What if people notice that I'm not making sense and I'm fired? What if I lose my mind?

Well guess what, when you're having a setback you have a chance to prove to yourself not only that there aren't any catastrophic events - but that you can even have a good day!

When things are going backwards, it is the time to take all focus away from sleep and shift it to the day. Find the reserves within and do something fun! Spoil yourself. Let yourself enjoy something you love.

This opportunity provided by a setback is your best chance of getting past sleep anxiety and becoming fearless. Because when you have a good day after little sleep, you see that you really have nothing to fear.

If you're getting better and better sleep by spending less time in bed and shifting attention towards pleasure, that's fantastic. If you on the other hand feel like you've taken a few steps backwards, then you're in luck.

Because you've made so much progress that you're in a place from which you can have a setback and you're in the midst of a unique opportunity to grow your sleep confidence, become fearless and sleep amazingly well for the rest of your life!

BE CAREFUL WHAT TO TELL YOUR FRiENDS

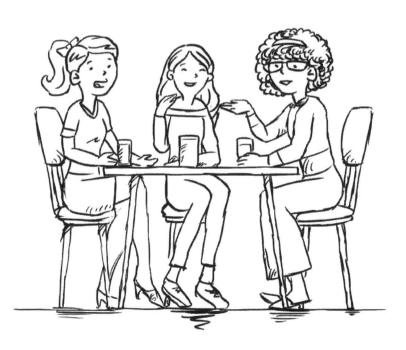

When you're in a tough spot, talking to a friend is almost always a good idea, because they have your back. You never have to wonder about what intent a friend or family member has, they're always thinking about what's best for you.

If you for example are trying to lose weight, a friend might tell you to join her spinning class. Great advice! If you're looking to buy a used car, your uncle can help decide which is a lemon and which is a fair deal.

When it comes to sleep, things are different. There are four reasons you should resist the urge to tell someone about what you're going through.

Firstly, they probably don't get it.

A friend that has never had trouble sleeping will not be able to understand what you're going through. They're confused and surprised and can't figure out how you can't sleep. Something they have no problem whatsoever with. That reaction in itself is a problem - it will make you feel as if something must be wrong with you, as if you have something really weird going on.

Secondly, when your friend goes on to tell you to worry less or take some melatonin, they're making things worse. Their true intent is for you to get better, but they don't realize that you cannot decide not to worry and that melatonin does not produce sleep. They're trying their best, but they just don't understand the problem and send you down a rabbit hole.

Thirdly, telling someone you have trouble sleeping affirms that you have a problem.

Although it does feel better once you've told a loved one how little you slept or how tired you are, it doesn't help you in the long run. Because saying out loud or in writing that you can't sleep makes it more tangible and real. Just talking about a problem like insomnia makes it bigger.

Finally, your near and dear may start identifying you as someone with trouble sleeping. They expect you not to sleep well. They start asking you about your sleep which brings attention to an issue that grows when it is put in focus.

So should you not talk about your sleep at all?

Absolutely not! When you have even the slightest positive to report, tell the entire world! Tell you friends, family members and random strangers that you slept really well yesterday and that you feel fabulously refreshed today.

That way you will not get any weird looks or friendly sleep tips and ever more importantly, you will affirm that you CAN sleep and that there's nothing wrong with you. And soon enough, those affirmations create a reality where you sleep amazingly well all the time!

THE ABILITY TO SLEEP

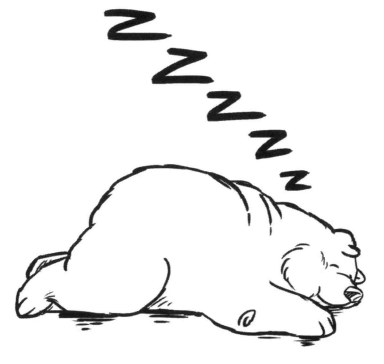

If you've been really worried about your sleep, you may have feared something eons of sleep has been lost over - losing the ability to sleep. There are few things you hear someone with insomnia worry more about. If you have, you're in good company.

Here's the thing, ability can mean two things when it comes to sleep. It can refer to your body's ability to produce the biological process called sleep and it can refer to your ability to make yourself sleep.

Whichever you have worried about, know that neither are possible to lose, but for very different reasons.

There are certain things without which we humans cannot survive. Consuming calories is one. Sleep is another. Let's add breathing for good measure. All of these are physiological functions that are indestructible. And although it may feel the opposite way, sleep is the one you need to worry about the least.

Although one cannot lose the ability to consume calories, you can keep yourself from eating to a point where you harm your body. Although you cannot lose the ability to breathe, your behaviors (like smoking) can lead to you having a lot of trouble breathing. Also, you could run out of food and be in a low oxygen environment, both which could be harmful.

Unlike food and oxygen, your body can produce sleep. You can never run out of sleep. If in short supply, your body can just make some more. It's like the central bank.

And just like the biological functions of calorie consumption and breathing, your body's ability to produce sleep is indestructible. In other words, you cannot lose your body's physiological capacity to produce sleep.

Now let's turn to that other way of looking at ability, the ability to put yourself to sleep. Can you lose that?

It may seem that way. When you struggle to sleep no matter what you do, and people around you have no such problems at all, it can seem like they have maintained an ability to sleep that you have lost.

But that's not what's happening.

Ask someone who sleeps great what they do to make themselves sleep and you'll just get a confused look.

They're not doing anything at all. In fact it is the complete lack of effort that makes them sleep so well.

It's not that you have lost an ability you had in the past that is the problem, it is that you've started to look at sleeping as a skill. A skill you never had.

You never had the ability to make yourself sleep, nobody does. It was the absence of effort, the absence of trying to produce sleep that had you catching all those Zzzs you're missing now.

You're on your way back to that place.

DON'T WAIT ANOTHER DAY

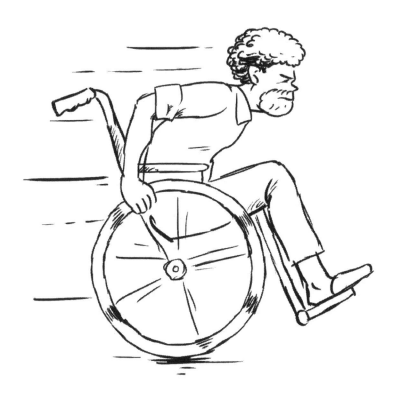

We are often told that we need to get a sufficient amount of good quality sleep in order to have the energy to do that thing. That thing you've wanted to do that insomnia has kept you from doing. Signing your kids up for skating classes. Learning to play the banjo. Visiting that friend in Singapore. There's been that thing you've just put off until you sleep better.

You have to do it now. Because whomever is telling you to wait got it all backwards. And that may include yourself. Here's why:

Firstly, great sleep happens when there's no effort. That person who always sleeps amazingly well does that because she is not trying at all. When you're keeping a mental list of things you will do when you're sleeping better, you're creating performance anxiety. Whether you'll do things that are enjoyable and meaningful depends on how well you sleep. Sleep becomes the gateway to a good life. Too much pressure.

Secondly, a great night follows a great day. And yes, you're more likely to have a great day if you had a great night. But which do you have most control over? That's right, you have much more control over what you do during the day. You can do things you enjoy even when you feel tired. When you have a better day and stay focused on something other than sleep, you have a better night. When you have a better night you'll have an even better day. You see where this is going.

Now if you do that thing today, that thing you've been putting off, you're proving that you can do anything you want even if you're not sleeping great. You're proving whomever is saying you can't wrong. That's always fun. But more importantly, you're showing yourself that sleeping a certain amount is not a requirement to enjoy life. And when there's less pressure, beautiful sleep happens.

DO YOU NEED A SLEEP DETOX

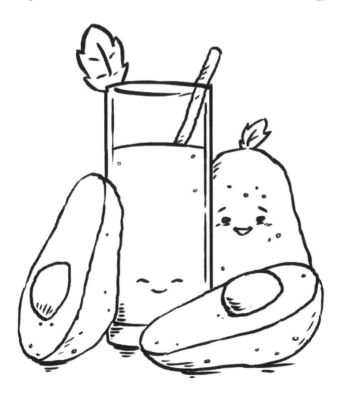

Getting to a place of sleeping well requires some learning. You have to understand why you're not sleeping well to have the motivation to change habits that are standing in your way. In addition to the learning you're doing here, you may follow sleep experts on social media or read articles and watch YouTube videos about sleep.

Here's the thing - learning is important, but you can have too much of a good thing.

Remember that insomnia is driven by attention. People who sleep great do that because they don't have a single thought about sleep in their brains. Someone who thinks of nothing but sleep on the other hand is all but guaranteed to have serious issues sleeping.

That's where a sleep detox comes in. This is an ideal approach for someone who feels that learning is not taking them any closer to sleeping fantastic. If this sounds familiar, you should seriously consider one.

Here's how you do it:

First, pick a time frame, 10 days or two weeks is a good starting point. Next, when your detox begins, you keep yourself from consuming any information at all related to sleep. No reading, no podcasts, no YouTube.

You may find after completing it that you've really started sleeping better. In this case you can extend your detox to get even more benefit. Don't be surprised if you find yourself extending it until it no longer is a thing. You're in a state of permanent detoxification. You've stopped worrying, caught a bunch of Zzzs and feel no need whatsoever to learn about sleep!

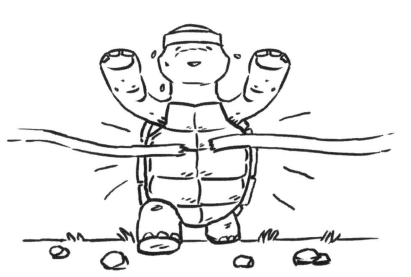

HOW TO PREPARE FOR A MARATHON

What would you tell someone who asked you what they should do to be prepared for a marathon they're running tomorrow? And yes, that's tomorrow in about 16 hours. And b78y the way, they haven't really done anything so far.

Chances are you won't really know what to respond. You'll probably be wondering how someone can think they can do something on the last day when they should have been training for weeks.

Sometimes it's hard to give someone the reality check they need - there's nothing you can do today that will prepare you for your race tomorrow.

This said, there are lots of things you can do to make things worse.

If you decide to run a half-marathon or do some intense calf work today, then you'll probably destroy your already slim chances of finishing that marathon tomorrow.

So what has marathon prepping got to do with sleep?

Quite a bit it turns out.

Imagine someone asking you what they should do the hour before they go to bed to sleep the best. That is exactly like asking what to do the day before a marathon. The hour before bed and the day before a long run both have minimal impact. It's too late to make any difference in a positive direction.

To be in good shape for a marathon, some 16-18 weeks of work is needed. To be in good shape for sleep, it all starts 16-18 hours before bedtime. Getting up at the same time and having an active day, now that makes a big positive difference!

Keep in mind that just like with running preparations, you can do a lot to sabotage your sleep the hour before bedtime. The main culprit is doing something that is aimed at making you sleep. Taking a hot bath that you hope will relax you enough to sleep, meditating so you become less anxious are examples of things that seem like a good idea but just make you focus on sleep. And the more you focus on sleep, particularly near bedtime, the more insomnia you will have.

Start your sleep prep early every day (but don't think of it as sleep prep, you're just as having a good day). Do things you enjoy that keep your thoughts away from sleep. And as for that last hour before you go to bed you already know what's most important - that you look forward to it!

ANTICIPATORY INSOMNIA

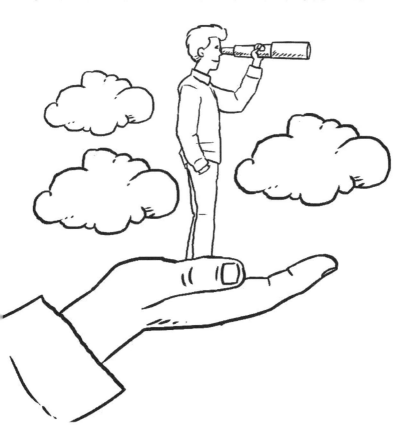

If you have trouble sleeping before a presentation or before traveling or the night before any other specific event, you have anticipatory insomnia. It's very common and here are some important things to be aware of that will help you get past it:

Firstly, sleeping less the night before anything of importance is normal. Think about when you were a kid and it was the night before Christmas. There were probably times when you were so excited that you just couldn't sleep. Having a job interview is no different. Your emotions are heightened to make sure you don't mess it up which does make you sleep less. However, the same hyperarousal also keeps you focused and sharp and helps you get that job. Sleep reduction ahead of a big day is completely normal, that's important to know so you don't start trying to avoid it and create the problem of anticipatory insomnia.

Secondly, even though you know in advance that you won't sleep well before that presentation, there's nothing you can do preemptively to make yourself sleep more that night. It's tempting to try to figure out things you can do ahead of the particular night when you anticipate not sleeping much. But all this does is build even more pressure and more focus on the night of, making it less likely still that you'll get a restful night.

If knowing that you can't take preventive action sounds disappointing, then think of it this way - by not trying, you're going to save yourself loads of frustration, preoccupation and sleeplessness.

Thirdly, you may be worsening your anticipatory insomnia by placing too much emphasis on how you sleep the night before an important event. For example, you may be thinking that if you don't get enough sleep, you will give a terrible presentation. And yes, it's true that if you sleep better you think better, but many other things influence your performance. Sleep is just one of many, many factors.

Here's what to do, look for evidence that sleep isn't that important. Remember that time you literally got 0 hours of sleep and still did fine or that other time when you slept lots and still had a no good day. Those are crucial pieces of evidence that everything does not hinge upon how you sleep. The more you work on changing your belief system and deemphasizing the importance of sleep before an event, the more Zzzs you'll catch.

Fourthly, you are doing yourself a big disfavor if you cancel the event. If you decide not to go on that trip because you think you'll have trouble sleeping, well then you've created proof that you can't sleep. Or so it may appear. The act of not doing something because you're afraid of losing sleep seems like evidence that there are things you can't do because of your insomnia. In reality, when you cancel an event you're canceling an opportunity to show yourself that you can do well even if you don't sleep much.

And you don't need a whole lot of counter evidence to make a big difference. One single time when you go on a trip you dreaded and find that you actually had fun is enough to remove the fear of travelling.

Use these insights to your favor, and you soon will not have more trouble sleeping before an important event than you should have!

ARE WE THERE YET?

If you've ever spent more than 30 minutes in a car with kids you will have heard the obligatory question of how much longer it will take. And not just once. It can seem like those little ones just don't have any patience whatsoever as they keep asking the same thing over and over again.

In reality, we adults aren't that different.

Just like young ones, we want to know what's happening. We want to know how long a flight will take, how long the wait is to see the dentist and when that package will arrive. What makes us seem more patient than kids is that we have a better perception of time. We know what two hours or 2 days feels like. And having that perception makes us feel even more in control when we know when something will happen.

We can live with having to wait 3 weeks, as long as we know that we will get that important haircut on March 3rd. Installing a new floor will take 2 months, no problem! As long as it gets done on time we're happy.

Knowing when something will happen takes away anxiety and is just very satisfying.

All this said, it is natural that you wonder when you will sleep well. Will it take 2 weeks, 2 months, more?

Just like when it comes to anything else, knowing what to expect is very desirable. But there's a big difference when it comes to getting to a place of amazing sleep and travelling to Hawaii - whether you wonder how long it will take does not actually affect how fast the airplane flies, but it does affect your sleep journey.

Here's the thing - insomnia is fueled by attention. The more you think about your sleep, the more preoccupied you become the less you get. The more you wonder how long until you sleep well, the longer it will take. When you count how long you've been trying to get to a place of good sleep and ask how many more days or weeks, you're taking steps away from your goal.

It's not easy, but try as much as you can to keep moving forward even though you don't know how long until you reach your destination. Directing your attention towards things that you enjoy will make the journey feel faster.

And when you do what you wish those kids in the car would, not ask how much longer until the destination, you will get there before you know it!

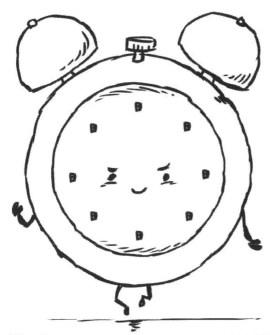

Have you ever stood over a pot of milk waiting for it to boil? If so, you know that it takes forever. Leave for a second on the other hand and you return to a burnt mess. Does this mean you have the power of speeding up time? Are you bending the laws of physics simply by leaving the kitchen?

Nope, that's not what's happening. What's bending here is not time but your perception of time.

If you think about it you can surely come up with many examples of when waiting for something to happen makes it feel like it takes a long time. Waiting for the bus, waiting for an important phone call, waiting for your kid to put their shoes on, you name it.

Waiting to fall asleep is no different.

When you go to bed waiting to fall asleep, your perception becomes skewed. 15 minutes of wakefulness feel like 45. 45 minutes feel like 2 hours. 2 hours feel like 4. 4 hours feel like you literally didn't sleep the entire night.

By the way, people that have no trouble sleeping have a lot of misperception as well. They overestimate how much they sleep at night by about one hour on average. Because they're not waiting for sleep to happen.

That's the direction you're wanting to move in.

But how do you do that?

Replace waiting with something you enjoy!

When you go to bed at night, you might want to read an interesting book. Or, you may want to watch a Netflix show that you've been thinking about all day. Anything that does not involve laying in a dark room waiting for sleep to happen is the way to go.

Similarly, when you wake up at night, it also helps to speed up time.

Taking a mental journey may be all you need. Or perhaps something creative? Perhaps listening to a podcast you like will work? Whatever you do, make sure it is something that you find pleasure in. Because if you pick a boring book or audiotape, then you will slooooow things dooooown again.

Change your perception of time and it will feel like you've changed the laws of reality.

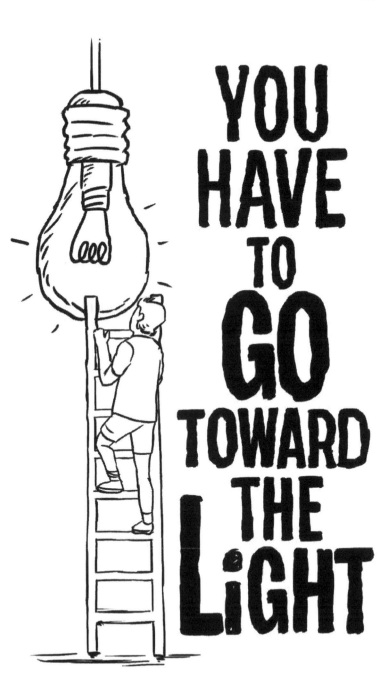

Something everyone with trouble sleeping has wondered at some point is which activities are helpful and which should be avoided. You may be surprised to hear that it's very easy to decide what you should and shouldn't do to get the best sleep - the answer depends entirely on the intent.

And finding your underlying intent is very straightforward.

Here's the thing - when we try to avoid any negative emotion or situation, things get worse.

When we do things to feel less sad, whatever action that is simply highlights that we are sad which produces more sadness. When we are anxious and try to avoid that feeling by whatever means, we become more anxious. Insomnia is no different.

When you go for a hike because you're not willing to have insomnia, the result becomes more sleeplessness. Because every step of the way you will be thinking about how your hike will affect your sleep. Preoccupation and self-monitoring become anxiety which produces more insomnia. What you tried to escape just became a bigger problem.

When you on the other hand do something for the simple reason that it sparks joy, or that it feels meaningful and gives you purpose, without a single thought about how it will affect your sleep, you're on the right path. You're no longer trying to get away from the dark, you're going towards the light.

Next time you wonder if you should or shouldn't do this particular thing, ask yourself what your intent is. If you see that you were planning to go to yoga class because you were hoping it would make you less anxious, not a good idea.

If you on the other hand find that you're wanting to go swimming because it's something you've always enjoyed and you look forward to - then suit up and jump in!

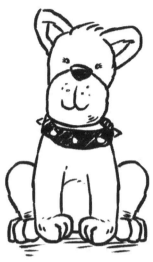

LET YOUR GUARD DOWN

When you are afraid of losing something, it is natural to start protecting it. And most of the time, this strategy makes sense.

If your bike is not locked, it's more likely that someone steals it. If you leave your phone unattended while ordering another coffee you might never see it again. When there's a risk of losing something tangible, it makes sense to guard it. Using a bike lock and keeping your phone with you not only is a good idea, it's a practical one. It works.

When it comes to losing sleep, things are very different.

It may appear that you are losing sleep to a mysterious villain. Guarding the sleep you have left therefore seems important. Getting that weighted blanket, the sleep mask and Valerian root extract will safeguard your sleep from the sleep thief.

But it doesn't work. He got past the security system and stole even more Zzzzs.

You need a stronger defense. Enter the Tylenol PM and the meditation app.

But no, the thief got past every safety stop and the worst part is, you know he'll be back for more.

Here's the thing though, there is no thief. Your fear of losing sleep is the culprit.

The behavior of protecting sleep creates a notion that you are at risk of loss. The behavior of guarding sleep creates a feeling that safekeeping is important. Your defense system creates the illusion of a burglar. The illusion of a burglar increases your fear of losing sleep. The fear creates more insomnia.

What you have to do, at least if you want to sleep better, is to dismantle your security system.

When you use a regular blanket and sleep no different, you realize the weighted one wasn't helping you. When you skip the Valerian root extract and don't see any changes in your sleep, you see that it didn't preserve your sleep.

Letting your guard down can feel like a scary proposition. But it's important, because that guard is the villain you thought it was protecting you from.

THE TWO TAILWINDS

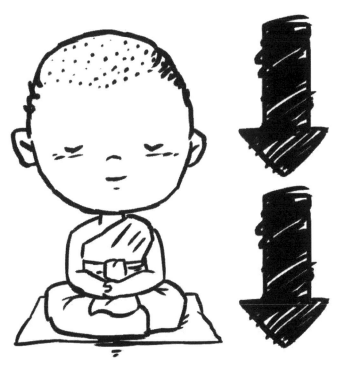

A very helpful concept form Buddhist philosophy is the two arrows. Briefly, it goes like this: The first arrow is an insult we can't avoid, like burning your lip on hot coffee. The second one is your reaction, scolding the barista. The second arrow is the one that hurts us the most and the one you can avoid.

Insomnia is driven by the second arrow - your reaction to sleepless nights that would have self-resolved without your attempt at trying to preserve sleep.

This said, you already know that. And we will not spend more time going over the two arrows analogy.

Rather, we want to focus on the opposite. The mirror analogy derived from the original, one we can call the two tailwinds.

Here's the thing - just as your reaction can turn a small problem into a ginormous one, your reaction can turn a small positive into a huge leap forward.

For example, if you find with Set it & Forget it that you fall asleep sooner than you expected one night, celebrate it! If you fall back asleep without a struggle another night, make it a big deal, share the good news, tell someone that you're sleeping better!

Sleeping better is a positive in itself, a breeze nudging you forward. Your strong positive reaction is the gush of air that will carry you miles closer to that place of peaceful sleep for the rest of your life.

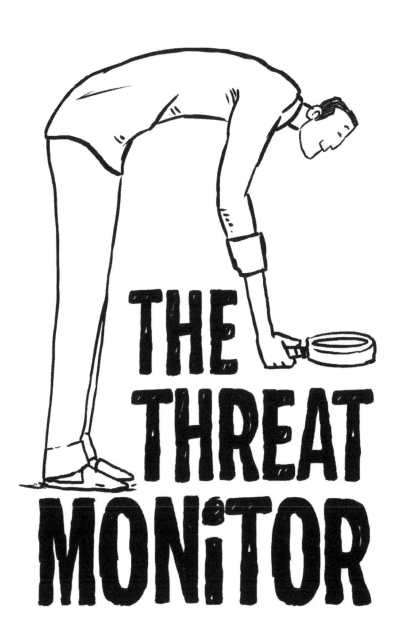

You should be very familiar at this time with why insomnia happens. We've looked at the three P model and you've heard about how your brain identifies insomnia as a threat.

But where does that reaction come from? Why is it that you become worried about not sleeping and start trying to do things to preserve sleep?

Here's the thing - like all humans you have a threat monitor in your brain. Some believe this is the amygdala, some that it is a more complex system that the amygdala is part of. Either way, it serves an important function: To keep you safe.

When you're crossing the street, your threat monitor makes sure there aren't any cars coming your way. When you notice that your tire pressures are low, your threat monitor will keep going off until you get that fixed. It will not see you hurt on its watch.

Having a threat monitor is the perfect mechanism for avoiding physical harm, but in a world with less tangible outside threats, it can get confused.

Insomnia happens when sleeplessness is identified as a threat, something that can hurt you and needs to be dealt with.

When it comes to a physical threat like a grizzly bear, it makes sense to educate yourself about bear behavior to make sure you're not hurt. This when it comes to a perceived threat like sleep loss translates to you reading up on the effects of sleep deprivation and insomnia.

When it comes to a physical threat it is practical to look for ways to fix it. This translates to you trying supplements or changes in your bedroom.

As there is no threat however, your threat monitor is not helping but hurting you. It creates an illusion that you are under attack and need to take measures to defend your sleep. This process increases anxiety, worsens insomnia and heightens the threat monitoring further.

So how to take sleeplessness off the threat monitoring radar?

The key is in the doing.

You cannot think yourself out. You cannot simply make a decision to stop threat monitoring. You have to do things every day that you enjoy and that keep you from even thinking about sleep.

When you start taking attention away, your threat monitor may initially become desperate, trying to keep you focused on the perceived problem that needs fixing,

This is your opportunity to train your brain.

Resist the urge to read up and experiment. Focus all your attention on something non sleep related that you enjoy. When you do, the threat monitor learns that there are no catastrophic events following sleepless nights even when you ignore it. It gradually turns off the alarm bells and keeps those quiet until there's a real reason to sound the alarm.

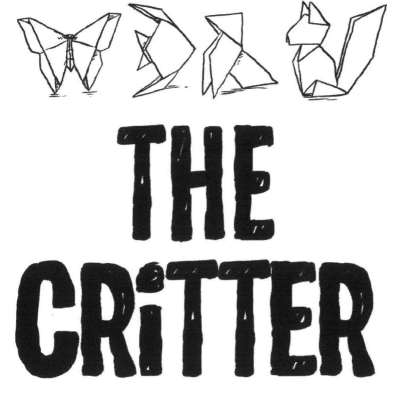

THE CRITTER

Although insomnia really is nothing but your brain's defense system identifying sleeplessness as a threat, it can be hard to put this knowledge into practical use. When this is the case, the analogy of insomnia being a critter can be really helpful.

Imagine a critter, something not well meaning but also not frightening. Something small and at this point mildly annoying. This is insomnia in the early stages.

The critter has certain preferred nourishment that makes it grow. As it grows it becomes more demanding as its appetite increases. If not fed regularly on the other hand, it shrinks and eventually disappears.

Here's the thing - the critter's diet is the key to making sure you're not feeding it. Or feeding it as little as possible. The three things it thrives on are the following:

Fear

Time

Attention

The more afraid you are of the critter, the stronger and bigger it grows. Like a bully, it feeds on you dreading what it will do to you. The more time you spend trying to appease it, the more influence it has over you. The more you try to figure out why it's there, and what you can do to get rid of it, the more powerful it gets.

Fear in this analogy is the fear of losing your sanity or having health problems because of insomnia. As we have seen, there is no evidence for this ever happening.

Time in the analogy is the time spent in bed trying to get more sleep. Attention is the effort of trying to understand why you can't sleep and what you can do to sleep more.

When you see that there is nothing to fear, that insomnia is completely harmless, when you start spending less time in bed and shift your attention in a different direction - the critter stops growing. In fact, it starts shrinking.

It may very well start acting up as you feed it less, an extinction burst is a positive sign, but as you keep not giving it any nourishment, it will eventually disappear.

OPENING THE SLEEP WINDOW

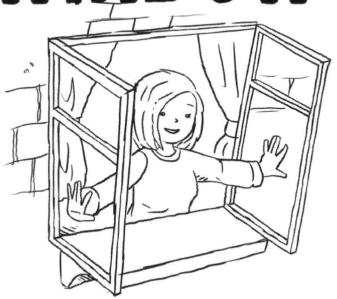

A common question from people that have begun their journey with Set it & Forget it is what to do if the pressure of sleeping within a tight window in itself produces insomnia. Or, at what point is it time to start going to bed earlier again.

Opening the sleep window can be the solution if this applies to you.

Let's look at an example to see what this means, how you can open your sleep window and if this is something you should do.

Jim has had trouble sleeping for a while and has decided to use a 6.5 hour sleep window from 11:30 pm to 6 am. Things are going really well and three weeks later he is sleeping pretty well. His sleep confidence is already improving and he's not very worried about sleep. He is wondering what his next step should be.

For Jim, a great move could be to decide to stop checking the time at 10:30 pm and then just go by how he feels. If he feels sleepy he goes to bed. If not he'll do something enjoyable until he does.

Jim has opened his sleep window. He keeps a consistent rise time at around 6 am but now has more flexibility on the evening side. This can help him sleep more as well as retraining himself to recognize cues for sleep.

Ana has also started using a sleep window but a 7 hour one. She is getting up at 6 am but is struggling to stay up until 11 pm. She frequently falls asleep at 8, 9 and 10 pm.

This is another scenario where not trying to stay awake until 11 pm but rather to 10 pm and after that not checking the time can be really helpful. Having an earlier but more realistic target time can make falling asleep at 8 or 9 pm more avoidable.

Thirdly, if you feel that only having let's say 7 hours allotted for sleep is anxiety producing, then not checking the time starting 8 hours before your rise time may work really well.

As always when you make any changes related to your sleep times, or if you do anything to improve your sleep, there can be a period of increased self monitoring. You're checking to see if for example opening the sleep window is going to have you sleep more or less. This self monitoring can often cause temporary increase in insomnia. If this happens, know that it's not a sign that your strategy is not working, just keep going and the dust will settle.

Having a sleep window is probably the most important and practical tool there is to get past insomnia. But sometimes a good strategy is to open up that window and let some refreshing sleep in!

GREED IS NOT GOOD

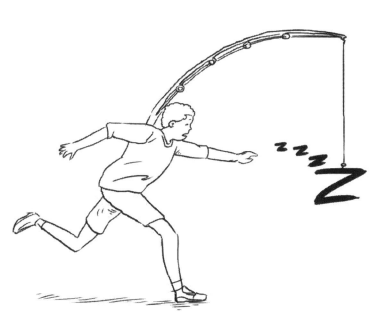

When it comes to many aspects of our lives, greed is a good thing. When it comes to money and power, maybe not. Wanting more from life itself on the other hand propels us to do things that are meaningful, fun and collaborative.

When it comes to sleep, there's no ambiguity. Greed is not good, neither when it comes to quantity or quality.

Greed for more quantity is often where insomnia starts.

Someone that had no problem sleeping but noticed that they're just getting 6.5 hours on average and wants to sleep more is a classic example. As we can't control how much we sleep trying to get more only leads to frustration. Frustration leads to trying even more which creates even more frustration and there you go with the insomnia spiral.

Greed for more quality is another common insomnia starting point.

This message is not for someone that has obvious troubles sleeping, you should want to improve your sleep quality! No, this is for someone that is feeling that sleep isn't refreshing anymore. There's no specific concern, you're sleeping fine, you're not snoring much, but you're just feeling tired. When this is the scenario, sleep is almost never the culprit, and trying to improve sleep quality when there's no obvious issue also leads down the insomnia rabbit hole.

The absence of greed on the other hand, perhaps we can call it contentment or acceptance, is a super power when it comes to sleep.

Use it every time you get a chance.

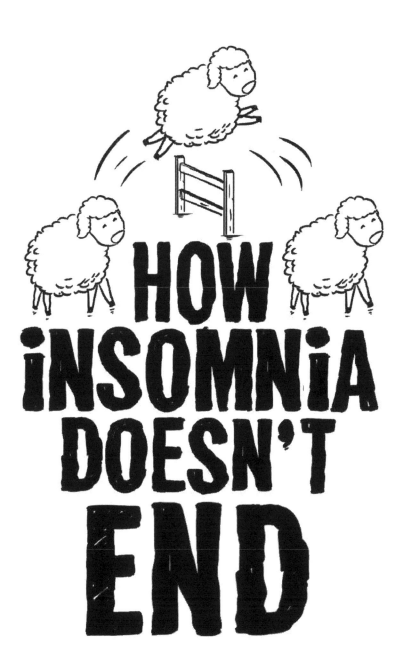

If you want to reach a goal, if you want to get to a certain place or destination, it can be very helpful to study previous travelers of the path you're on. You can learn a lot from what made their journey successful, but it is equally important to learn what turned out to be a dead end.

Or worse yet, a trip to the land of Oz.

"After years of searching, I found Milkweed, this herbal supplement grown in the Himalayas, and now my insomnia is history". Says no real person ever.

You may hear this type of language in an ad or affiliate marketing post but never from someone who got past years of insomnia. The reality is, the quest to sleep better never ends with finding that one supplement, medication or gadget. Years of searching the internet for a remedy that will end the battle in bed does not lead to you discovering "the thing".

Rather, the process of trying to find something that will work for you gives insomnia its oxygen - attention. Whether in the form of preoccupation, anticipation, self monitoring, experimentation or any other way you spend time on sleep, you give insomnia the attention that keeps it alive.

Now check this out - realizing that the quest to sleep better and the search for a remedy has been fueling your insomnia all this time IS "the thing".

This realization is the discovery of the path that leads away from searching, away from struggling and towards a place of sleeping peacefully forever.

HOW INSOMNIA ENDS

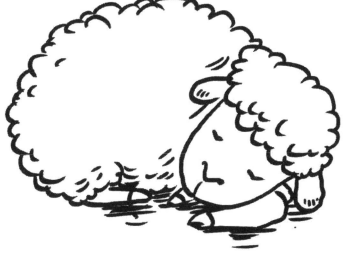

Whenever someone no longer has trouble sleeping, it is a great opportunity to ask what helped and what didn't. Both are really important to know when on the path towards sleeping well. What didn't help is often the most important. Knowing about the dead ends helps you avoid them. This is why we have already talked about the rabbit holes and the search for "the thing".

Just a hair behind in importance comes the insights and habit changes that do lead you past insomnia. And the one thing you hear from virtually every single person is a version of:

I stopped worrying.

I stopped worrying is consistently the most common answer you get from someone that no longer has trouble sleeping. This is no surprise as worrying about sleep almost always is what drives insomnia. And if worrying is no longer in the picture, neither is insomnia. But this insight begs a question - how do you stop worrying?

Here's the thing, you can't decide to stop worrying. This only leads to more attention given to worrying, more time spent thinking about worrying and more worries.

The answer is in understanding and doing.

It may not seem like you have control over what you think and feel. But you do. Because emotions come from thoughts and you can change your thoughts with education. In fact, your thoughts about sleep have probably already changed. And you may already have noted that you are less anxious because of the changes in how you think about sleep.

We also have control over what we do. And when you change what you do you reinforce the helpful new ways you started thinking about sleep.

More specifically when it comes to sleep, the doing consists of spending less time in bed and doing things that are fun during the day.

Besides "I stopped worrying" common things people say made a big difference is not trying to figure it out and caring less about how much one sleeps. These are basically variations of worrying less. When you're less worried you spend less time trying to figure out why you have trouble sleeping and you're less preoccupied with how much you sleep.

Not worrying about sleep is how insomnia ends. And the key to not worrying is changing how you think and what you do. Educate yourself, spend less time in bed and do things daytime that you enjoy and that shift your attention away from sleep. Set it & Forget it.

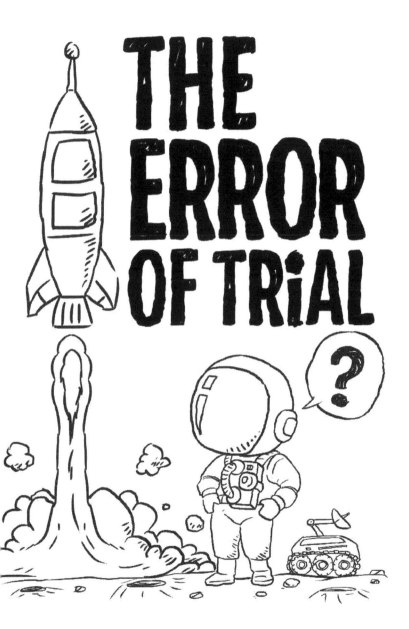

A strategy that works for almost any problem is to try a bunch of approaches, dismiss any that doesn't seem to work and keep going until you find the solution. Trial and error is super practical and can be done with no or minimal supervision.

When it comes to trouble sleeping however, trial and error is all but guaranteed to make things much, much worse.

Here's the thing - insomnia is not caused by lack of efforts. Quite the opposite, it's a result of problem solving. It is the process of trying to figure out why you can't sleep and what you should do to sleep more that is the root problem.

A person that sleeps fantastic does that because they have not a single thought about sleep in their minds. Which by the way is very different from "shutting your mind off", nobody can do that. Those great sleepers sleep amazingly well because they exert 0 effort trying to sleep more or better. The complete lack of attention focused in this direction is why they have no problems sleeping.

Trial and error doesn't work when the problem you are trying to solve is your problem solving.

That's the main reason not to apply this otherwise amazing tool when it comes to difficulties sleeping.

The other reason is that trial and error can become a speed bump even when you're on the right track.

Let's say you've started spending less time in bed to get better quality sleep. 10 days later you're not sure the strategy is working. You've had a few better nights but lots of sleepless ones too. You're wondering if you should continue.

In many circumstances, it makes perfect sense to do what you're doing: Evaluate your method to see if you should keep going or abandon it. In fact abandoning any strategy that doesn't work quickly is the reason trial and error is so effective.

The problem is that it can take a while before you start seeing that Set it & Forget it works. And self-evaluation gives insomnia attention which is it's oxygen. You may abandon a great strategy for a reason that is totally valid when it comes to anything but sleeping better.

So what to do?

As much as you want to make sure you're on the right track, try the Set it & Forget it approach. Learn, change habits and other than that, try not to question whether it was the right call, if you should do something else or if it will work for you.

Because when you're no longer problem solving, the problem of problem solving no longer exists.

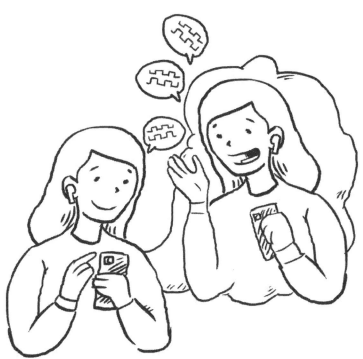

TELL YOURSELF WHAT YOU NEED TO HEAR

Affirmations are like the force, very powerful and have two sides. The dark side is affirming negatives, telling people that you can't sleep for example. The bright side is to affirm positives. Starting to use the bright side will give you unlimited momentum on your path towards sleeping fantastic.

Before we get practical, let's spend a second on the power of affirmations. Let's do an imaginary experiment. Think of something you believe is false, "kale is delicious" or "I can't stand chocolate" for example. Now imagine that you would repeat this out loud some 20 times, tell a friend and text another for good measure. At the end of the day, guess what you would feel about what you've echoed all day? That it's actually true. Or at least more true than it seemed before you started affirming it. Now imagine what happens to your belief in your own ability to sleep when you start affirming that you can sleep.

Here's the thing - telling yourself that you are six feet tall is not going to change your stature, because it has nothing to do with confidence. How well we sleep on the other hand has everything to do with confidence.

Try asking someone that has no trouble sleeping what they do to sleep. You'll just get a confused look. Even the thought of doing something to sleep is completely alien to someone that has solid sleep confidence. Affirmations can take you a long way towards being that person.

What you should start doing today is actively look for positive signs that you can affirm. If you feel those are few and far between, that may be because you haven't looked hard enough. Seek and you shall find.

And remember, even a hint, a whiff or a notion that something is going your way is all you need!

Let's say you fell asleep a bit sooner than you expected one night. Perfect, go affirm! Say out loud that you fell asleep faster than you thought you would. Tell a friend or two. If you're working with a sleep coach or therapist, share it with them as well.

If you're noting that you feel pretty refreshed on a day you didn't think you would, make it a big deal! Write it down. Do something to celebrate. Give it all your attention.

When you start affirming positives, you're strengthening your belief in yourself, in your own ability to sleep, your sleep confidence. You're using the bright side of the force of affirmations.

If you keep it up you will reach a place where if asked what you do to sleep, you will find the question odd. You don't do anything in particular. Then you'll remember that time you had trouble sleeping and tell the person asking you about the power of affirmations.

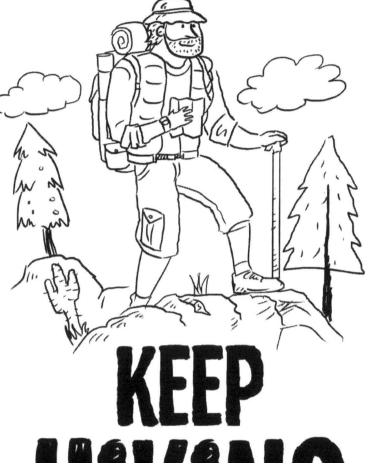

One of the most common questions from people that have started using Set it & Forget it is - what do I do when it's not working?

This could be someone who did better initially but then had a night of sleeping almost nothing. It can be someone who has limited time in bed for 3 weeks and hasn't noticed any changes. Or someone who feels they've hit a plateau after some improvement.

Here's the thing - when you have trouble sleeping, you want to solve that problem. But the attempts at trying to solve it ends up being what keeps sleeplessness going. The instinct when nothing is happening or you've had a setback is to tweak things, change direction or try something different. But the best thing to do is the opposite - stay the path.

A really good way to think about this is to imagine yourself hiking up to a mountain top. At the summit is a place of really good sleep.

As you are making your way up, you are very likely to stumble on a root or a rock. That's expected. If you stop and examine the root that made you trip, if you wonder why it happened, why it is sitting there and how you can avoid this happening again, you'll never reach the top. You'll get stuck at that root.

If you just keep hiking on the other hand, you will get there.

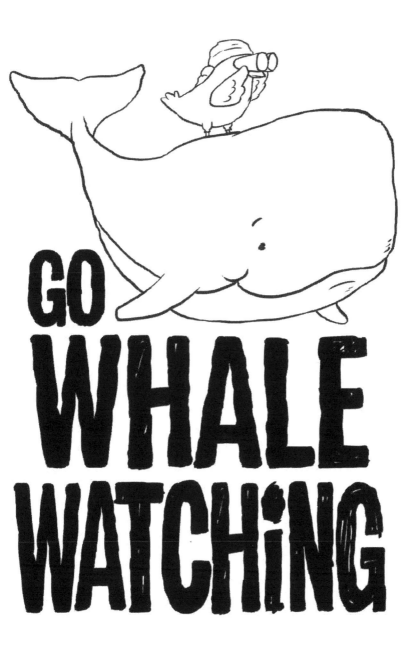

When we have a problem - we want to solve it. Nothing surprising about that. A strategy that almost always is the right one.

Got a leaky faucet - call the plumber. Annoying headache take some ibuprofen. Can't find the car keys - figure out where you most likely put them and look there.

For most problems, the solution lies in taking action and/or figuring out what caused it so that can be addressed.

With insomnia, things are different. It is the process of trying to fix the problem that maintains the problem. To solve it, you have to use a strategy that may go against all your emotions and instincts...

....go whale watching!

When you do something enjoyable like taking in the spectacle of huge water living mammals migrating up the coast, you step away from trying to sleep, wanting to sleep and trying to figure out why you're not sleeping.

Behavioral activation is the technical term for doing stuff you enjoy. If not whale watching then perhaps baking, synchronized diving or yoga is your thing. It really doesn't matter as long as your attention shifts away from sleep.

Attention is oxygen for insomnia. It cannot survive without us thinking about it, trying to do things to sleep and studying our sleeplessness.

Get that behavioral activation going, leave the insomnia without oxygen, and sleep better forever!

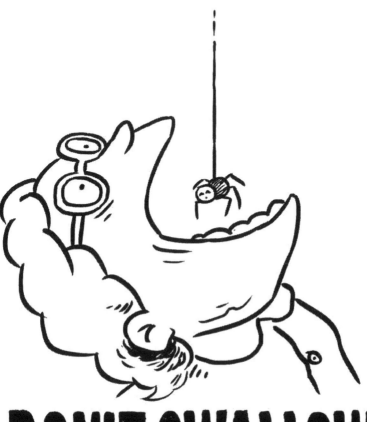

Are you familiar with the children's book about an old lady who swallowed a spider? If so you can skip this next paragraph. If not, here's how the story goes:

An old lady randomly swallows a fly. To get rid of the fly she swallows a spider. To get rid of the spider she swallows a bird. She goes on to swallow increasingly large animals until she finally downs a horse and collapses.

There are two really important learning points from this story.

Firstly, swallowing a fly is not a disaster.

Nobody wants to swallow an insect. Just the thought makes you nauseated. However, it's not a terrible ordeal either. If you can just get over the fact that it happened, the problem becomes self-limiting. It's an issue that would have resolved by itself if left alone.

Secondly, increasing efforts means increasing problems.

The downhill spiral didn't start with swallowing a fly, but a spider. The old lady could not have avoided the first, random event. The more she tried to get herself to unswallow the fly however, the worse off she got.

So what has this got to do with sleep?

Here's the thing - we swallow flies all the time. We go through days or weeks of stress during which we sleep little every so often. If we don't go on to look for a spider to ingest, things get back to normal.

Now you may think that it's a little too late for this analogy to help you. Perhaps you've already swallowed a bird or even a dog. Guess what - everything you read here will help you get good sleep no matter how far down the path of trying to get that fly you've gone. There's nothing you've done that cannot be undone.

The real take home message here though is that there will be many flies coming your way, and you will swallow several.

You will have a night or a stretch of nights when you sleep very little. You'll have days when you feel unrefreshed and foggy. You will feel an urge to do something, take a sleep aid, buy a weighted blanket, sleep in a different room.

When you're looking to do something like that to fix your sleep issue, remember the old lady who swallowed a fly. That will keep you from doing what got her into such a mess - swallowing a spider.

REACT
TO THE
GOOD

As humans we are hardwired to look for things that aren't right and ignore things that are working well. From an evolutionary standpoint it makes perfect sense to focus on any potential threat. Any problem that can lead to our destruction needs to be dealt with to increase our chances of survival. The problem is that we no longer live as hunter gatherers in a hostile environment and our wiring often trips us up.

When your spouse forgets to put the dishes in the dishwasher, you take note of that. You find it annoying that you have to remind her again to do what everyone else does. When she on the other hand does fill the dishwasher four consecutive days, you don't feel in a celebratory mood and overwhelm her with praise. She's just doing what she's supposed to do.

We react to problems and let the absence of problems pass us by, making us feel there are plenty of issues and few confetti moments in our lives.

When it comes to sleep things are no different.

If you wake up early and don't fall back asleep for a long time, this triggers you to wonder what happened and maybe complain to a coworker. If you don't wake up on the other hand, you don't give your office manager a high five and tell all your siblings. As you can imagine, reacting only to negatives can make it seem as if nothing good ever happens in your sleep world. And in a world of doom and gloom, great sleep rarely happens. The prophecy has fulfilled itself.

This is why you have to train your brain to do the opposite of what it's wired to do: React to the absence of a problem and put all those red flags back in the closet.

In practical terms, here's what you need to do: When you slept well for one night and had 2 sleepless ones, then react to the good one. Spend a lot of time thinking about how well you slept that time. How refreshed you felt when you woke up. How easily you drifted off. If you had one day when you felt refreshed during a week of being drained and foggy - tell everyone willing to listen about how amazingly well you felt that day.

You won't notice an immediate change, but if you keep going, if you keep training your brain to see the good, it will start to automatically pick up on positives rather than problems. And when that happens, how you perceive your sleep will completely change. You will be presented with an increasingly rosy picture in which you don't have any issues sleeping.

And guess what, when it comes to a problem like insomnia, which is driven by our thoughts and beliefs, reality is only one step behind perception.

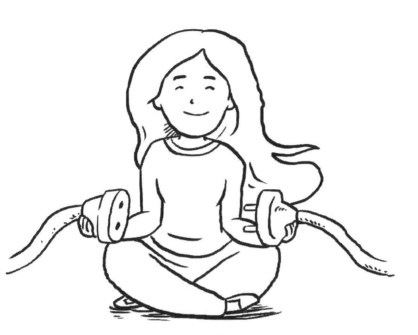

Have you ever been sold to by a salesperson who was desperate for you to buy their product? Someone who's life seemed to depend on you making an instant purchase? If so, ask yourself if their behavior made you more or less likely to look for your credit card or the exit sign.

You probably went for the latter. You felt pushed in one direction and went the other. The sales person made a big mistake, they were too attached to the outcome.

Let's go into some depth here and explore the psychology of sales because we can learn a lot that applies to sleep. The key question being: Why don't you want to buy from someone who desperately wants to sell?

Here's the thing - you want to make a purchase when there's no pressure. When you're allowed to make a decision that is best for you and the person you're buying from seems to have your best interest in mind.

When you on the other hand feel manipulated and pressured to open up your wallet, you hold on tighter. Your spidey senses are going off and you feel a need to make sure you're not losing money.

Now imagine that you're selling sleep to your brain.

Your position is that sleep is important because so much depends on how you sleep. Your ability to function, your happiness, your health and your well being. Your brain on the other hand is looking at loss of sleep as a threat. It is doing everything it can to keep you from losing sleep. Or so it thinks.

Where it is confused is in not realizing that sleep is a passive process. That it cannot happen as long as it acts as if losing sleep is a threat. And here's where the negotiating comes in:

If you tell your brain that it's really important you get some sleep because you have a big presentation tomorrow, what you're really asking is that it loosens up, dials down the threat monitoring and allows you to sleep. You're pressuring your brain to relax.

Well guess what, when you suggest letting go, your brain, thinking letting go means giving up on keeping you safe, balks. The mere suggestion signals that you're not serious about safety and that it has to tighten the grip on sleep further. Needless to say, more insomnia is coming your way.

Just like the salesperson, being attached to the outcome has gotten you the opposite results of that which you want.

The learning point - detach yourself from the outcome and magic will happen.

Just like a great sales person is thinking first and foremost about you, giving you all the space and time you need, not making you feel pressured or manipulated, so you should approach your sleep.

Find evidence that you can do just fine on little sleep. Prove to yourself that plenty of other things affect how you feel during the day. Tell your brain sleep isn't that important.

When you detach yourself from the outcome, you're giving your brain permission and freedom to de-escalate. To stop trying so hard to keep you safe, to loosen its grip on sleep and to be less cautious.

And when that happens, you will get the outcome you wanted in the first place - that peaceful, refreshing sleep you deserve!

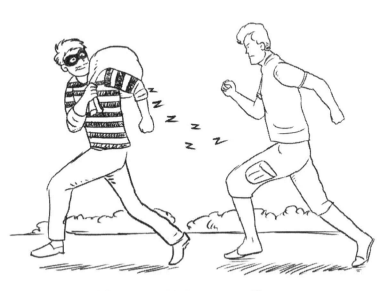

Imagine two people living in the same neighborhood. Samuel is very cautious and lives next door to Sara who has a very laid back attitude. They both hear that someone had a package stolen from the curb on the very street where they live just a few days ago.

Sara doesn't think much of it. She continues not to lock her front door and believes the stolen package may have been taken by accident or that there's some other benign explanation for what happened.

Samuel on the other hand has been thinking about safety for a while and decides to download a neighborhood app where he can stay informed about what's happening in the vicinity. He also installs a video surveillance system.

Sure enough, just a few days later Samuel notices when reviewing the recordings that an unfamiliar man went all the way up to his front door but didn't ring the doorbell. Also, he learns from his app that others have seen similar things on their surveillance cameras.

Samuel's behavior confirms that his decision to beef up security was the right one. He has already found evidence that there are things going on that he needs to be aware of. Sara on the other hand is equally pleased with her decision not to change her behavior. She continues to feel like nothing is going on.

Here's the teaching point - Samuel's behavior of threat monitoring builds a belief that there are threats he should monitor. Things he is doing to stay safe makes him feel there is something he should stay safe from. Looking for potential problems creates the illusion that there are problems he should look out for.

When it comes to tangible physical threats like burglars, you can argue that taking safety precautions are important to minimize your risk of harm. Or you can argue that the negative impact on your mental well being from threat monitoring outweighs the potential benefit of avoiding a break in. Both sides can make good points.

However, when it comes to sleep, there is no physical threat. Sleeplessness is a perceived threat. Therefore, the act of threat monitoring only has downsides.

When you read about how insomnia affects your health, it creates a belief that losing sleep affects your health. When you track your sleep, you start feeling like keeping track is important. In reality, all you're doing is making yourself believe that there is a problem and that it needs to be monitored. And that's definitely hurting your sleep.

Be like Sara. Know that looking for a thief creates the notion that there is a thief you should look for. Know that if a problem only exists when created by your thoughts and habits, it disappears when your belief system changes. And not doing anything that makes you believe in a problem is a big step toward a place where that problem no longer exists.

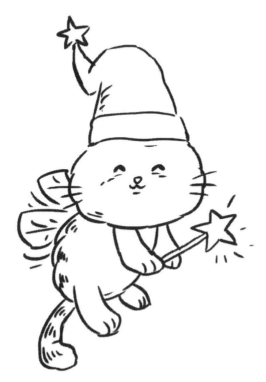

MAGICAL THINKING

When uncle Joe puts his Yankee cap backwards and stands on one leg to make that home run happen he's engaged in something called magical thinking. He believes that his actions can influence something that in reality will or will not happen no matter how he wears his cap or how he stands. What uncle Joe does is common and harmless. In fact, it can even be fun. Both for Joe who enjoys the sport even more as well as for friends and family who get to tease him!

When it comes to insomnia on the other hand, magical thinking is never helpful and often part of the problem.

Let's say that you drink some hot milk every night at 8 pm hoping it will keep you asleep. As milk cannot produce sleep, this is an example of magical thinking. You're doing something that in reality has no influence whatsoever over the thing you want to influence.

So why is drinking hot milk not harmless and fun just like standing on one leg?

Here's the thing, uncle Joe's behavior does not shake the confidence of the Yankee's lineup. None of the players will ever believe that if Joe just had stood on the other leg, they would have gotten that home run. If they did, that would become a serious problem. Because instead of focusing where it matters, literally keeping their eyes on the ball, they would be looking into rituals and superstitions and start losing games.

Your behavior of drinking hot milk on the other hand does have a big impact on how you sleep. The milk itself is a non factor, the belief that it influences sleep on the other hand isn't.

If you have some hot milk and coincidentally sleep well your sleep confidence is hurt because you're starting to believe in rituals and superstitions. For a while it may seem like you're better off, but the next time you're sleepless, you start wondering why the milk "isn't working". You modify your ritual by drinking it later or you add another one like wearing a sleep mask. You're going deeper down the rabbit hole.

If you have some hot milk and sleep no better then you end up frustrated that nothing is working. Best case scenario you abandon your ritual and don't replace it. Chances are however that you look for another magical way of producing sleep that leaves you even more frustrated.

If knowing that you can't use magic to produce sleep makes you disappointed, think of it this way - you've just saved yourself months, perhaps years of confusion and frustration. And guess what, when you start sleeping amazing without any rituals, superstitions or potions, it will feel like magic!

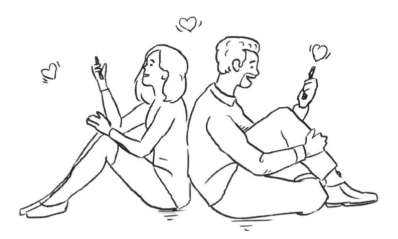

PLAY HARD TO GET

There may be no more classic move in the dating playbook than playing hard to get. The objective with this behavior is to make someone desire that which they can't have. It's similar to the psychology of time limited sales and temporary offers that exploit your scarcity mindset. The greater the risk of missing out on something, the more we just have to have it.

If you're not convinced that playing hard to get works, then imagine the opposite - someone desperately wanting you to want them. Imagine that you're on a date with someone and it becomes clear during the first minutes that they're way ahead of you. They're already picturing you married, naming your future children and planning family vacations. Even if your date has some great qualities, their desire to make it work will suffocate any romantic feelings that you may have developed.

Insomnia has it figured out. Big time. In fact, you would be challenged to find anyone that plays this game better.

It may start gradually with you getting a bit less and less sleep over weeks. You wonder what's happening and day by day become more afraid of losing something you thought you had. Or it may start out of the blue with a series of completely sleepless nights and you're hooked immediately. You so want that sleep you're not getting.

Here's the thing - you mustn't fall for it! The more you're wanting the sleep that has become so elusive, the less of it you'll get. Your desire to sleep will suffocate any possibility of sleep happening.

In fact, you have to do the opposite: Play the game even better than insomnia.

Go to bed later and get up earlier. Pay sleep no attention. Look the other way. Flirt with any activity you're interested in!

Keep going and inevitably sleep will fall for you. Because that's what happens when you master the art of playing hard to get.

THE BEGINNING

I sincerely hope that this book has been helpful to you. I hope that it has made sense and that this is the beginning of a new chapter for you. One in which you don't struggle with sleep and live your best life.

If you still have questions, head over to the YouTube channel and leave a comment. Or visit The Sleep Coach School online and use the form to submit a question to be answered in an Open class episode.

Thank you again for giving me a chance to help you sleep better!

/Daniel

Made in the USA
Middletown, DE
03 September 2021